AN ARITHMETICAL AND MEDICAL ANALYSIS OF THE DISEASES AND MORTALITY OF THE HUMAN SPECIES

PIONEERS OF DEMOGRAPHY

A series of collective reprints of the more important milestones in the development of historical demography.

THIS SERIES INCLUDES:

The earliest classics: John Graunt and Gregory King
Mortality in pre-industrial times: the contemporary verdict
Enclosure and population
The population of Ireland before the 19th century
Population and disease in early industrial England
Comparative statistics in the 19th century
Slum conditions in London and Dublin
Mortality in mid 19th century Britain
Rates of mortality
J.-B. Bertrand: *A historical relation of the plague at Marseilles in the year 1720*
T. Short: *Comparative history of the increase and decrease of mankind*
T. Short: *New observations on city, town and country bills of mortality*
W. Black: *An arithmetical and medical analysis of the diseases and mortality of the human species*
E. H. Greenhow: *Papers relating to the sanitary state of the people of England* (General Board of Health Papers)

Each volume contains a new introduction.

William Black

AN ARITHMETICAL AND MEDICAL ANALYSIS

OF THE

DISEASES AND MORTALITY OF THE HUMAN SPECIES

LONDON 1789

With an introduction

by

D. V. GLASS

1973

GREGG INTERNATIONAL PUBLISHERS LIMITED

ISBN 0 576 53286 X

Printed in Germany

INTRODUCTION

D. V. Glass

Though the name of William Black is usually mentioned in discussions of the history of medical statistics, it is by way of illustration of the development of the subject as such rather than as a contributor of particular distinction.[1)] The entry in the *Dictionary of National Biography* is not untypical in that respect. 'Black did not attain any remarkable eminence in his profession, but wrote some books which are not without value as illustrating the application of the statistical method to medicine'. Nor is this somewhat muted comment entirely unfair. There is nothing in Black's work comparable to the great initial jump of John Graunt, whose *Observations* were remarkable not only in representing an entirely new development—there was no earlier model to emulate or improve upon—but also in their contributions to methodology. Graunt showed the kinds of questions which had to be asked of statistics on cause mortality, and especially of defective statistics; and perhaps even more remarkable, he formulated the concept of the life table, basic to all modern mortality analysis and applicable to many other fields of inquiry. Black could scarcely have repeated that kind of performance. At the same time, given the data available in the 18th century—defective records of christenings and deaths in London—he could not undertake the kinds of analysis possible in the latter half of the 19th century. By that time William Farr had built up, with the co-operation of the medical profession, a body of cause mortality statistics which, though by no means perfect, nevertheless permitted studies of the highest relevance for socio-medical policy. The contributions of Black were inevitably more modest. Nevertheless they deserve to be remembered, and not simply for reasons of antiquarian interest.

William Black (1749–1829) was born in Ireland and obtained his medical training in Leyden, where he received the M.D. in 1772. He became a Licentiate of the Royal College of Physicians in 1787. He practised in London, living in Piccadilly, and appears to have been associated with Sir Gilbert Blane in the General Dispensary for Poor Married Women.[2] After retiring, he died in Hammersmith in December 1829, in his eightieth year.[3] He must have been impressed by the ravages of smallpox in London, for his first publication on medical statistics, *Observations Medical and Political, on the Small-Pox, and the Advantages and Disadvantages of General Inoculation, especially in the Cities* (London 1781; a second, enlarged edition was published in the same year) dealt in some detail with that disease. But studying smallpox mortality no doubt awakened an interest in mortality statistics in general, for even in that publication considerable attention is given to the broader subject and also to the defects in the London Bills of Mortality, which formed the basis of much of his analysis. Subsequently he wrote on the history of medicine and on insanity, his work on this latter subject again coming within the field of medical statistics and being based upon a study of cases in Bedlam—an extension of the tables in his *Arithmetical and Medical Analysis*. But his most comprehensive study of medical statistics was the book reprinted here, *An Arithmetical and Medical Analysis of the Diseases and Mortality of the Human Species*. First published in 1788, and originating in a lecture he had been invited to give to the Medical Society of London, it was withdrawn by Black before the edition was sold out and was replaced by a second edition, 'corrected and enlarged', in 1789. (It would seem, however, that the new edition was prepared somewhat hurriedly, for towards the end of the volume the author explains that he had omitted some fifty additional pages of comments on causes of death.) It is this second edition which is now reprinted.

The book falls into two parts of unequal length. The first, consisting of the two initial chapters and a final chapter on the Bills of Mortality, provides a general demographic background; the second and much larger section is more specifically medical and deals with individual diseases. The demographic section, which, for obvious reasons, I find particularly interesting, presents an estimate of the population of the world and its continents, and an estimate of the age composition of the population of Europe. Then follows a discussion of such matters as age at puberty, age at marriage in Britain, urban-rural differences in marriage and fertility, and the sex ratio at birth. The discussion is based largely on the work of the standard authors of the 17th and 18th centuries, with whose writings Black was obviously very well acquainted. Political arithmeticians, early demographers and medical statisticians are covered—ranging from Petty, Graunt and Davenant (in effect, of course, Gregory King, whose estimates Davenant cited), through Huygens, Halley, Jurin, De Moivre, Thomas Short, Süssmilch, Richard Price and even Muret. Thus the estimate of the age structure of the population of Europe represents—as Black admits—a simple application of Davenant's estimate for England and Wales, in turn derived from Gregory King, whose work was not published in full until 1804. I have suggested elsewhere that King's estimate was probably not too unrealistic, though it overstated the proportion of the population aged 60 years and over.[4] King's estimate was made at the end of the 17th century, since which time mortality had very probably fallen. (Black himself stated that mortality from fevers had decreased, plague had been eliminated, scurvy had become insignificant as a cause of death, and the numbers of murders had diminished, though those of suicides had increased). But mortality has much less influence than fertility on age composition. For Europe as a whole it is not unlikely that fertility was higher than in England and Wales, if only because age at marriage was lower in the Eastern and South Eastern regions. If the expectation of life at birth was around 30 years and if on the average a woman surviving to the end of the childbearing period had around 6 live births, then the 'stable' age structure would have consisted of about 41 per cent under 15 years of age, 55 per cent between 15 and 60, and 4 per cent 60 years and over.[5] This would be a somewhat younger population than that depicted by Black—and with only half of his proportion aged 60 years and over—but not too radically different. And it is this very large proportion under 15 years of age, as well as the high death rates in infancy and childhood, which would have accounted for the dominance of infant and child deaths in the total picture of mortality. Black drew attention to the fact that, according to the London Bills of Mortality, there were more deaths under 2 years of age than between the ages of 2 and 40 and he later argued that acute diseases of infants and children under 2 accounted for almost a third of the total deaths in London. The real picture may well have been even more striking, for the Bills of Mortality were incomplete in their coverage and probably especially defective for the youngest infants—those who died within the first few days after their birth. In London in 1849, when mortality was still very high but when the vital statistics were very much more reliable (civil vital registration had come into force in 1837), deaths under 2 years of age did not form quite so large a proportion, but they were still almost as numerous as deaths between 2 and 29 years. And deaths under 5 years of age were almost 25 per cent more numerous than deaths between 5 and 39 years.

Black's estimate of the population of the world and its regions is—perhaps surprisingly—worthy of consideration. It must have been arrived at after inspecting earlier attempts, judging from Black's comment that these showed enormous variation. But his figures differ considerably from those of such pioneer estimators as Riccioli, Vossius and Süssmilch. Further, in contrast to those earlier figures, Black's results agree surprisingly well with modern estimates, which, though no doubt very imperfect, are at least based upon a much greater expertise in handling poor demographic data than could have been applied in the 18th century. For example, take Carr-Saunders' revision of the estimates of Willcox, and compare his figures with those of Black. As Table 1 shows, the comparison is by no means a ludicrous one, especially bearing in mind the fact that Black drew attention to the uncertainty of his statistics, which might, he said, err by between 100 and 300 millions. He was in any case highly sceptical of most of the methods currently used to estimate population and well aware of the defects in the data on which they were based.

Table 1. Estimates of World Population (in millions).

	(a) Black	(b) Carr-Saunders	
Year:	1789	1750	1800
Europe	130	140	187
Americas	20	12	25
Africa	150	95	90
Asia	500	479	602
Oceania	—	2	2
World	800	728	906

Source: A. M. Carr-Saunders, *World Population*, Oxford 1936, p. 42. The Willcox estimates are given in W. F. Willcox, 'Increase in the population of the earth and of the continents since 1650', in W. F. Willcox, ed., *International Migrations*, Vol. 2., New York 1931 (reprinted New York-Princeton-Paris 1969).

In his introductory discussion of mortality, Black had one advantage over John Graunt, namely that from 1728 onwards the London Bills of Mortality reported ages at death, though not in combination with causes. Graunt had had to infer the likely level of infant and early childhood mortality from the causes of death as such—that is, by assuming that certain causes applied wholly or largely to infancy. Black, by contrast, had the reported ages, though they were subject to errors and omissions. (He believed that the number of burials should be increased by 25 per cent to allow for omissions.) It was these statistics which formed the basis of the comment mentioned earlier (on high mortality in the first two years of life), as well as of his statement that half of human mortality occurred during the first 5 years of life and that in the metropolitan centres of Europe half of the children died before their third birthday. What the situation was when Black was writing, we still do not know with any precision. But though mortality was extremely high, it is probable that these figures overstated it, for they were based upon the kind of technique used by Richard Price in constructing his life tables from absolute numbers of deaths (without relating the deaths to the populations in the corresponding age groups). This technique is appropriate only when the population is, and has long been, stationary, with an unchanging mortality. With a growing population, the technique overestimates mortality, as the Government discovered later after selling annuities for premiums based upon Price's famous (and erroneous) Northampton life table.[6]

If we use a correct life table technique, and assume that the expectation of life at birth was around 30 years, then out of 100 live born babies about 37 would die by their fifth birthday and about 56 would die by the age of 30 years. To match Black's estimate of 50 per cent dying by their fifth birthday would involve an expectation of life at birth of only about 20 years—the kind of level which might have obtained in epidemic situations in underdeveloped societies before the use of modern insecticides and antibiotics.[7] In India in the period 1911–21, a period during which the 1918–19 influenza pandemic attacked undernourished and malnourished populations, expectation of life at birth may well have fallen to that low level.[8] It is still a matter of speculation whether so low an expectation of life obtained in London in the late 18th century; for England and Wales as a whole the level was more likely to have been around 30 years or even somewhat higher. In the 1840's it was around 40 years for males and 42 years for females; for London in that period the reported figures were around 35 years for males and 38 years for females. Since then, the situation has changed radically, and developments in the 20th century have resulted in a reversal of the relative positions of London and England and Wales, as well as in almost a doubling of life expectation in London. In 1966, the figures were 68·4 years for males and 74·7 years for females in England and Wales; for London the figures were about 69·1 and 76·3 years.[9]

One last item in Black's demographic introduction is worth noting—his reference to longevity. Though he referred to some of the apocryphal cases of extreme longevity, he was justly sceptical of customary mythology. He believed that 70 to 80 years was the upper limit for most of mankind and that it had been so since the days of Moses. Longevity is not incompatible with a low overall expectation of life at birth; and it has sometimes been argued that, with high general mortality, the selection process may give rise to cases of great longevity. Black, however, doubted whether among the 4 million deaths per year, which was his estimate for Europe as a whole (which would have yielded the unrealistically low crude death rate of about 31 per 1000), there were as many as 2000 deaths above the age of 100 years. This would mean a ratio of 0·5 per 1000 deaths; in England and Wales in 1966 the ratio was 0·8 per 1000, for deaths at ages 100 and over, in spite of the much older population and the much higher life expectation. Of course, a higher expectation at birth does not necessarily mean an increase in the span of life and in fact the great reduction in mortality achieved during the past 150 years has been in respect of mortality before old age rather than during it. Errors at the older ages in the 19th century and changes in the basis of life table construction since the first official life table for England and Wales make it hazardous to attempt to be precise in documenting the extension of extreme old age. But the official life table for 1961—for which, especially because of pension and other requirements, the order of accuracy at advanced ages is likely to be quite high—records a probability of survival for males from birth to the age of 100 of only 0·7 in a 1000, and for females of 2·6 in a 1000. (For those who have attained age 60, the probability of continuing to live until 100 would be 0·86 in a 1000 for males and 3·04 in a 1000 for females). These results are derived from current life tables—that is from tables based upon the age-specific death rates observed in a limited period of time, namely 1960–62.[10)] A very valuable alternative approach to the study of old age mortality has been developed by Vincent.[11)] This, which he terms the 'method of extinct generations', consists of cumulating deaths above a given age by both sex and calendar year of birth. The number of survivors of a specified age from a particular generation will be equal to the sum of all the deaths after that age of members of the particular generation. Several countries have tabulated deaths both by age and by calendar year of birth and work on four such countries—France,

Sweden, the Netherlands and Switzerland—for the period up to 1948 suggested that the differences in mortality rates between men and women diminish at the very high ages and become negligible above 100. Further, the shape of the curve of mortality suggested that, for the periods and countries studied, the limit of the span of life would be reached at about 110 years both for men and women.

It should, however, be remembered that the oldest men and women alive today were born at a time when the hazards of infancy and childhood were still very great—when infant mortality, for example, was around 150–160 per 1000. Moreover, the differences in conditions of life between rich and poor were extreme, especially in the growing urban communities. Black believed that 'the indigent and laborious class of mankind do not attain to longevity in the same proportion with the middling and more opulent ranks'. This contention was still regarded as debatable in the early 19th century, though the work of William Farr confirmed the existence of widely different levels of mortality of men in different occupations, while the later studies of T. H. C. Stevenson showed that the mortality rates of men, married women and infants were strongly associated with differences in their socio-economic position.[12)] And so far as the 19th century itself is concerned, Hollingsworth's research into the demography of the British peerage demonstrated the very wide gap in the expectation of life at birth between the peers' children born in 1825–49 and the children of the population at large born in 1840–41: for boys, the contrast was between 52 and 40 years; for girls, between 58 and 43 years.[13)] Analyses of death rates by period of birth, rather than by period of observation—that is, generation mortality rates—were pioneered by Derrick in 1926 and revealed a parallelism between the curves for successive generations, suggesting, in contrast to the views expressed by some 19th century physicians, that children brought up in periods of high death rates carry high mortality with them throughout their lives, though the curves are cut across by exceptional circumstances which affect most ages, such as influenza epidemics.[14)] Whether the children brought up in the environment of the very light infant and childhood mortality of today will show a much higher probability of becoming centenarians, only time will tell.[15)]

With the exception of the final chapter, which will be referred to subsequently, the remaining and far larger part of Black's book is focussed on specific diseases and naturally reflects the state of medical knowledge of the period. But Black belonged to the more advanced and constructively imaginative physicians of the period and this is evident in his discussions of the relative importance of different causes of death, in his attempts to estimate case fatality, in his criticism of the not infrequent nosological absurdities and confusions in the London Bills of Mortality and in his efforts to supplement those data by drawing upon the records of dispensaries in London and Newcastle. He was an advocate of inoculation (variolation), but realised that, to have any significant effect on smallpox mortality, inoculation would have to be done in infancy or early childhood. Hence his criticism of the London smallpox hospital which, he claimed, inoculated no one under the age of 7 years. In addition, in contrast to the author of a recent study of inoculation in Britain,[16)] Black believed that the numbers inoculated had been relatively small. 'Even in the London small-pox hospital, since its first institution, forty years ago, there have not been inoculated altogether 25,000'. He stressed the importance of 'consumption' as a cause of death, especially among the poor and more particularly among those living in cities. Between one fifth and one sixth of all deaths in the London Bills were from that cause (Table 2 suggests that in London in 1849 tuberculosis accounted for about one eighth of all deaths). And just as Graunt had carried out a special 'field study' to evaluate the reported deaths from syphilis, Black undertook a special study to estimate the number of executions, on which the London Bills were 'shamefully erroneous and defective'. He could find no records in London for the years prior to 1754, but was able to arrive at a 'reasonable' estimate for the period 1762–77, during which there had been some 1020 executions in London, 19 out of 20 being males and predominantly between 18 and 40 years of age. For Great Britain and Ireland as a whole he believed that the number would have been two or three times that for London, and that five or six times that total had been transported overseas.

Black knew that his statistical studies left much to be desired. Both in the final chapter of *Arithmetical and Medical Analysis of Diseases and Mortality*, and still more in the postscript to his earlier publication, *Observations Medical and Political, on the Small-Pox* (London 1781), he discussed the need for reliable and comprehensive vital statistics and the means of achieving them. Like Corbyn Morris in 1751[17)], and George Man Burrows in 1818[18)], he wanted much greater detail to be recorded at death registration—sex, marital condition, age (the first month of life to be shown separately, and the first year to be split into two or three periods; by single years up to age 5 and in 5 or 10 year age groups thereafter), disease and cause of death and how long the sufferer had been afflicted, as well as information on miscarriages and stillbirths, on the degree of maturity of the foetus and whether it had died during the process of childbirth. He urged that death registration be placed in the hands of medical inspectors—surgeons or apothecaries—paid initially £60 per year, but to be raised subsequently to £100—and that the classification and analysis of the data be entrusted to a medical superintendent, an 'able physician', with a salary of £200 per year. These recommendations had no immediate effect. But they helped to inform the medical profession of the importance of providing realistic data on mortality and of the practicability of improving the information on cause of death. With such recommendations from respected practitioners, it is not surprising that when the Select Committee on Parochial Registration was set up in 1833 to consider the whole question of vital registration, the Provincial Medical Association—the forerunner of the British Medical Association—submitted a resolution that cause of death be included in death registration.[19)] In turn, it was with the co-operation of the medical profession that Britain became a pioneer in the development of reasonably reliable cause mortality statistics. By that time, one of the causes which had contributed heavily to mortality in the latter half of the 18th century, and especially in London—smallpox—had lost most of its importance. But infectious diseases generally were still dominant. As may be seen from Table 2, they accounted for over 40 per cent of all deaths in London in 1849, a year in which cholera killed more than 14,000 people, about 20 per cent of all deaths in that year; if tuberculosis were included, the proportion would be raised to over 50 per cent. And even later, in the period 1848–72 in England and Wales as a whole, infectious diseases and tuberculosis together accounted for about a third of all deaths.[20)]

Table 2. Proportionate mortality: Deaths from specified causes as a percentage of deaths from all causes.

	London 1849[1)]		England & Wales 1848–72	
	Males	Females	Males	Females
Infectious diseases (excluding tuberculosis)[2)]	43·3	44·9	17·5	18·3
Tuberculosis (all forms)	14.0	12.1	14·6	15·5
Bronchitis and pneumonia	10·3	9·6	12·3	11·3
Other Causes	32·4	33·4	55·6	54·9
All Causes	100·0	100·0	100·0	100·0

1) The London data suffer from 'residence errors'. It was not until 1911 that births and deaths were transferred back to place of usual residence.
2) Deaths from convulsions under age 5 have been included for 1849. They were very largely concentrated in the first two years of life and were probably associated mainly with infantile diarrhoea. They are not so included in 1848–72, for they could not be distinguished in the overall statistics given in the source referred to below. But in that period infantile convulsions still accounted for almost a fifth of all infant deaths.

Source: London 1849: *Twelfth Annual Report of the Registrar-General of Births, Deaths, and Marriages in England*, London 1853, pp. 252–257. England and Wales, 1848–72: W. P. D. Logan, 'Mortality in England and Wales from 1848 to 1947' *Population Studies*, Vol. 4, September 1950, pp. 138–139.

1. See, for example, M. Greenwood, *Some British Pioneers of Social Medicine*, London 1948, p. 25; and G. Rosen 'Problems in the application of statistical analysis to questions of health: 1700–1800', *Bult. Hist. Med.;* 29, 1955, pp. 27–45.
2. According to H. R. Spencer, *The History of British Midwifery from 1650 to 1800*, London 1927.

3. I have not been able to find any biographical information more detailed than that given in the entry in the *Dictionary of National Biography*. The probate records in Somerset House (Askew and Abbot, January 1830) list only one William Black who died in Hammersmith at the end of 1829 or beginning of 1830. If this was Dr. William Black, he died a bachelor and intestate, his estate (assessed at £1500) passing to a widowed sister, his only next of kin.
4. 'Two papers on Gregory King', in D. V. Glass and D. E. C. Eversley, eds., *Population in History*, London 1965.
5. United Nations, *The Aging of Populations and its Economic and Social Implications*, New York 1956, pp. 56–57.
6. See William Farr's examination of the Northampton life table in the *Eighth Report of the Registrar-General*, London 1849 (reprinted in *The Development of Population Statistics*, Gregg International Publishers, Farnborough Hants England 1973).
7. United Nations, *Methods of Population Projections by Sex and Age*, New York 1956, pp. 78–79, presents the survivorship rates based upon a series of model life tables.
8. See Kingsley Davis, *The Population of India and Pakistan*, Princeton N.J., 1951, pp. 237–289. Davis estimates the deaths in India during the influenza pandemic at around 20 millions.
9. See my note on 'Some indicators of differences between urban and rural mortality in England and Wales and Scotland', *Population Studies*, Vol. 17, March 1964.
   The figures for 1966 are approximate—there was undoubtedly underenumeration of the population of London in the 1966 Sample Census—but cannot be far from the truth.
10. *The Registrar General's Decennial Supplement, England and Wales, 1961: Life Tables*, London 1968, pp. 26–29.
11. P. Vincent, 'La mortalité des vieillards', *Population*, Vol. 6, April–June 1951.
12. Farr's classic analysis was in the Supplement to the *Thirty-fifth Annual Report of the Registrar-General*, London 1875. For Stevenson's work on infant mortality, see *Seventy-fourth Annual Report of the Registrar-General*, London 1913. The analysis of the mortality of married women by the socio-economic status of their husbands was undertaken in connection with the 1931 census.
13. T. H. Hollingsworth, *The Demography of the British Peerage*, Supplement to *Population Studies*, Vol. 18, November 1964, pp. 56–59.
14. The generation approach to the study of mortality was first put forward in V. P. A. Derrick, 'Observations on (1) errors of age in the population statistics of England and Wales, and (2) the changes in mortality indicated by the national records', *Journal of the Institute of Actuaries*, July 1927. The idea of a generation life table is, of course, much older.
15. A recent actuarial study suggests that 'the shape of the mortality curve at age

80 and over is now being materially influenced by the proportion of the less hardy whose lives have been prolonged by favourable circumstances'. See E. A. Law and F. Seltzer, 'Uses of the life table in public health', *Milbank Memorial Fund Quarterly*, Vol. 48, No. 4, October 1970, Part 2, p. 27.
16. P. E. Razzell, 'Population change in eighteenth-century England. A reinterpretation', *Economic History Review*, Vol. 18, August 1965.
17. [Corbyn Morris], *Observations on the Past Growth and Present State of the City of London*, London 1751.
18. G. Man Burrows, *Strictures on the Uses and Defects of Parish Registers and Bills of Mortality*, London 1818 (reprinted in *The Development of Population Statistics*, Gregg International Publishers, Farnborough Hants England 1973).
19. *Report of the Select Committee on Parochial Registration*, London 1833, p. 174.
20. For a discussion of the continuing impact of infectious diseases (including tuberculosis) in England and Wales up to the 1920's, see B. Benjamin, 'Statistics and epidemiology', *The Scientific Basis of Medicine Annual Reviews 1972*.

THE MEDICAL WORKS OF DR. WILLIAM BLACK

1. *Observations Medical and Political, on the Small-Pox and Inoculation and on the Decrease of Mankind at every Age, with a Comparative View of the Diseases most fatal to London during Ninety Years*, London 1781.
   2nd edn. London 1782 (with changed sub-title.... *Small-Pox, and the Advantages and Disadvantages of General Inoculation, especially in Cities; and on the Mortality of Mankind at every Age in City and Country.*)
2. *An Historical Sketch of Medicine and Surgery, from their Origin to the Present Time; and of the Principal Authors, Discoveries, Improvements, Imperfections and Errors*, London 1782.
3. *A Comparative View of the Mortality of the Human Species, at all Ages; and of the Diseases and Casualties by which they are Destroyed or Annoyed*, London 1788.
   2nd edn., London 1789 (re-titled: *An Arithmetical and Medical Analysis of the Diseases and Mortality of the Human Species.*)
4. *A Dissertation on Insanity, Illustrated with Tables, and Extracted from between Two and Three Thousand Cases in Bedlam*, London 1810.
   2nd edn., London 1811.

AN

ANALYSIS

OF

DISEASES AND MORTALITY.

AN ARITHMETICAL AND MEDICAL ANALYSIS OF THE DISEASES AND MORTALITY OF THE HUMAN SPECIES.

BY WILLIAM BLACK, M.D.
ONE OF THE ROYAL COLLEGE OF PHYSICIANS IN LONDON;
MEMBER OF SEVERAL LITERARY SOCIETIES, &c.

PUBLISHED AT THE UNANIMOUS REQUEST OF THE MEDICAL SOCIETY OF LONDON.

THE SECOND EDITION, CORRECTED AND IMPROVED.

LONDON:
PRINTED FOR THE AUTHOR BY JOHN CROWDER;
AND
SOLD BY C. DILLY, IN THE POULTRY.

M.DCC.LXXXIX.

Reproduced by kind permission of the Royal Society of Medicine from a copy in their possession

Publisher's Note

Owing to technical difficulties the folding table facing page 42 has been reset

Republished in 1973 by Gregg International Publishers Limited
Westmead, Farnborough, Hants., England

TO HIS

ROYAL HIGHNESS

GEORGE

PRINCE OF WALES.

MAY IT PLEASE YOUR ROYAL HIGHNESS,

I HAVE the honour to lay at your Royal Highneſs's feet the ſecond edition of a Medical and Political Treatiſe, which your Royal Highneſs was moſt graciouſly pleaſed to permit me to publiſh under your auguſt patronage. Incited by the diſtinguiſhed honour of your Royal Highneſs's countenance, and by its favourable reception from the publick, I have endeavoured to render the preſent edition leſs unworthy of your protection. Reſpecting that malady in particular, which lately occaſioned ſuch affliction to your Royal Highneſs, and family, and to the nation, I truſt it will not be arrogant in me to ſay, there will be found conſiderable original, uſeful, and authentick information. I beg leave, moreover, to conclude with this ſummary obſervation, which I pledge myſelf, in the ſequel, to demonſtrate, both in the groſs, and in detail, by incontrovertible proof, that of the four millions of deaths, which I have calculated annually to enſue in Europe, one million of theſe might be annually preſerved, which are now prematurely ſwept away by various diſeaſes and caſualties; beſides, a ſtill greater number that might,

might, without much difficulty or expence, be added to the annual population. I ſhall prove, that the rudiments of the knowledge herein inculcated are not eſſential to the phyſician only, but are equally indiſpenſible to the Prince, the Stateſman, the Legiſlator, and the General, who are ambitious of pre-eminence and permanent renown.

I have the honour to remain,

With profound reſpect and eſteem

Your Royal Highneſs's dutiful,

And obedient ſervant,

WILLIAM BLACK.

London,
June 30, 1789.

CONTENTS AND INDEX.

INTRODUCTION.

INTRODUCTION.

ABOUT one century only has elapſed ſince the firſt introduction and analyſis of bills of births and mortality, in order to aſcertain arithmetically the value of lives and annuities; and it forms a moſt intereſting epoch in politicks, commerce, philoſophy, and medicine. The proſpects of life and death are calculated with the ſame exactneſs as the chances on dice, or the blanks and prizes in a lottery wheel. This ſcience, however, had been employed merely for the purpoſes of politicks and traffick; none of the ſyſtematick medical authors, to the preſent day, having ever converted it to the advantage of their own profeſſion, and of the community, medicinally. I believe the firſt dawn of medical arithmetick, in illuſtration of diſeaſes, will be found in Dr. Jurin, and was the laſt reſource in ſupport of inoculation, then in its infancy, but vilified in print by phyſicians and divines. It was by demonſtrating in numbers the comparative ſucceſs under inoculation, and the natural diſeaſe, that this inveterate conſpiracy againſt the practice could be defeated. Since that time, ſeveral fragments of medical arithmetick are difperfed in the mifcellaneous writings of Dr. Short. It has alfo been profecuted with indefatigable induftry by Dr. Robinfon of the navy, and Dr. Millar of London, on the fubject of fevers, in various parts of the globe, and the comparative fuccefs by different febrile remedies.

Thofe who are acquainted with the hiftory of arts and fciences, will not be furprized at the rancorous oppofition againft medical arithmetick. Such has been the fate and firft reception of many other ufeful difcoveries, and of the moft enlightened reformers and benefactors of mankind. The medical profeffion alone furnifhes us with many hundred proofs of this malignity of human nature, this confederacy of knavery and ignorance. The circulation of the blood, and the Peruvian bark had each thefe hoftile combinations and perfecutions to encounter. With refpect to medical arithmetick, what time muft yet revolve before ignorance and bigotry fhall be enlightened, prejudices and inveterate habits done away, envy, malevolence, and calumny filenced, I cannot determine.

Of this I am convinced, that it would be a moft fortunate circumftance for medicine and mankind, to whofe benefit the profeffion fhould be fubfervient, were the parliament of Great Britain to examine phyficians on every difeafe, as they have lately done on the unfortunate malady of a Great Perfonage. The utility of the arithmetical fyftem would then be as univerfally confpicuous throughout every difeafe, in any great emergency, as it was in infanity, or as it is in politicks and commerce. Various

reafons

reaſons of delicacy reſtrain me from touching upon that examination, except ſo far as the principles then adopted by the moſt exalted and wiſe men of the nation, or probably of Europe, in ſearch of information, are decidedly in approbation of the arithmetical ſyſtem. Throughout that examination, numerical data, in preference to the opinions, profeſſional doctrines, and jarring aphoriſms of auguries and oracles, were repeatedly called for: but it ſo happened, that mine, in the preceding edition of this work, were the only data of this deſcription ever publiſhed on the diſeaſe. And it was not a little flattering, that the interrogatories, in this national dilemma, to ſome of the medical ſuperintendants of Bedlam, were anſwered by a reference to my calculations. I was at the ſame time honoured with letters and viſits, on the ſame ſubject, from ſeveral of the firſt perſonages in the kingdom in rank and talents. A medical ſociety, diſtinguiſhed both for the number and literature of its members, had likewiſe previouſly ſtamped my labours, though then in an immature ſtate, with their warmeſt approbation.

But I truſt it is not neceſſary to ſhelter myſelf behind authorities or commendations, however dignified in rank and ſcience. In defence of the arithmetical ſyſtem, and heretical innovation which I have endeavoured to incorporate with medicine, I ſolicit no more than a fair trial, enlightened judges, and an impartial verdict, according to the evidence and merits. I flatter myſelf, that I ſhall be able, by its aſſiſtance, to refute the aſſertion of a great Orator in parliament, immediately after the ſecond examination of the phyſicians on the diſeaſe of a Great Perſonage; which was, "that medicine is a conjectural ſcience, and inſanity, above all other diſeaſes, the moſt conjectural in the ſcience." Without numerical data, there is too much truth in Mr. Fox's detection and expoſure of medical penury and ignominy, which is not ſingular, nor new. But that diſeaſe, which, above all others, is univerſally thought the moſt difficult and conjectural, I have particularly ſingled out, both on account of its importance at this extraordinary criſis, and to prove the immenſe utility and extent of medical arithmetick; and, in this inſtance, to put it to the moſt ſevere teſt and trial. In this and other diſeaſes I have broken open ſeveral fountains of truth and medical knowledge, which had lain concealed.

The great utility of medical arithmetick was an accidental diſcovery, at leaſt to me, about eight year's ago: for in the courſe of many preceding years attendance on medical lectures, at different univerſities, I never once heard the ſubject mentioned. I then found in London a violent literary warfare, reſpecting the advantages and diſadvantages of general inoculation, eſpecially in cities. Dr. Jurin had left half the buſineſs undone. For if, according to Baron Dimſdale, the principal opponent, inoculation in cities and towns, by ſpreading the natural infection, was likely, on the whole, to do more injury than benefit, policy and humanity would dictate the total ſuppreſſion of the practice. In conſequence of the Baron's publications, a cha-

rity,

rity, then inſtituted for general inoculation, was blighted: he had, in his opinion, triumphed over all his opponents: a few months, however, after the publication of my animadverſions on his different books, eſſays, and pamphlets on inoculation, he precipitately obliterated, in a new edition, the principles which he had maintained from his firſt appearance in print, in order to adopt my ſentiments. I cannot commend the motives as liberal which inſtigated the Baron to conceal the name of the author, to whom he ſtood indebted for his information, and of which I can eaſily convict him by indubitable teſtimony and proof.

That learned phyſician Dr. Arbuthnot, in his preface to Huygens, "de ratiociniis in ludo aleæ," ſays, "There are few things which we know which are not capable of a mathematical demonſtration; and when they are not, it is a ſign the knowledge of them is extremely ſmall and confuſed; and when a mathematical reaſon can be had, it is as great a folly to make uſe of any other, as to grope for a thing in the dark, when you have a candle ſtanding by you."

The analyſis, on an arithmetical plan of the public regiſters, not only of births, burials, and diſeaſes, but likewiſe of the collected records of hoſpitals, diſpenſaries, and individuals, are overlooked by all the modern ſyſtematick authors. They leave us equally ignorant of the aggregate, or comparative number, or the force of thoſe fiends which haunt and ravage the globe. To ſpeak metaphorically, in medical books, the extenſive deſolation of the moſt rapacious tyrants and conquerors are confounded with the uninterefting hiftory and petty depredations of a robber. The profeffors of medicine hitherto have been combating enemies, without afcertaining their comparative number or devaftation. Mr. Sauvages, a celebrated modern French writer, thus expreffes himfelf, "Utinam numerus refpectivus diverforum morborum a noftratibus inquirarentur." It is principally from ignorance on this fubject, fo ftrongly recommended by Sauvages, that far too many of the ftreams of medical inveftigations, and publications, of academick rudiments in medical knowledge, aud of various charitable donations to poverty in difeafe, have not yet been pointedly directed to publick utility.

Every one knows, that from his prognofticks, which are confined principally to fevers, the father of medicine, Hippocrates, was idolized in Greece, and is revered by pofterity. I am aware of the imputation of herefy, in calling the aphoriftick prognofticks contracted and pinioned. Without medical arithmetick it is impoffible to reach the "grandeur of generality," the fublime of medical divination. In order to form general propofitions of the ratio of mortality at various ages, and as influenced by climate, local fituation, diet, drink, luxuries, cuftoms, manners, profeffions, &c. of the abfolute and relative havock by different difeafes; and as influenced by age, caufe, and duration of the malady, together with the moft fuccefsful modes of cure, we fhould extend our views far beyond the narrow bounds of a parifh, or even of a province; we fhould include an interval of

many

many years, collective numbers, large groupes of mankind, and of morbid cafes.

Without difmembering prognofticks I could not exclude the caufes of difeafes. Indeed, diagnofticks, caufes, and prognofticks, conftitute more than one half, and the moft difficult of therapeuticks. Formulæ and recipes are the eafieft part; but I have not here propofed to treat of the Materia Medica. It was neceffary, in treating of morbid prognofticks, not only to afcertain the general danger, the abfolute and comparative mortality by different difeafes, but likewife to enter into more minute detail, and to meafure the proportions of cures, incurables, and deaths, and the various periods of time at which different difeafes ufually prove moft fatal. I have corrected feveral errors of preceding calculators and commentators on the general profpects and decrement of life; and I hope the malice of criticifm cannot juftly accufe me of arrogance, in faying, that I have greatly enlarged the fphere of calculation in a morbid ftate, by embodying a multitude of new facts, and reducing the whole into fyftem.

Again, when opinions are litigated in either medicine or furgery, and a thoufand different leaders hoift their feparate ftandards, affigning different caufes, prognofticks, and modes of cure, what tribunal can poffibly decide truth in this clafh of contradictory affertions and conjectures; or by what clue can medical wanderers find their way through the labyrinth of prognofticks and therapeuticks, except by medical arithmetick and numbers? Perhaps fome would here anfwer, the beft authors fhould decide the con-

controverſy. Who are they, ancient or modern; of what nation, univerſity, metropolis, party, or ſect? To borrow Moliere's ſatirical expreſſion, Hippocrates often ſays Yes, and Galen flatly No. The ſyſtem of medical arithmetick, although it may not ſhew the beſt mode of cure that may hereafter be invented, it will, however, by compariſon, determine the beſt that has yet been diſcovered, or in uſe. By this criterion we ſhould prove our ſuperiority over the phyſicians of the Continent. For as to our ſuperiority or excellence, even if founded in the collateral branches of general ſcience, it is of no conſequence to the community. Phyſicians have been too long running aſtray in ſpeculative or frivolous employments of philoſophick drudgery. They can ſcarce yet be ſaid to have liberated themſelves from the reins and fetters of ancient or of modern metaphyſicks.

Medical arithmetick eſtabliſhes on a ſolid foundation a multitude of the fundamental principles, or primary orders, of medical architecture; and erects platforms for compleating the entire ſuperſtructure. The lumber and mountain of ponderous ſyſtems heaped together from Galen down to Stahl, can only be compared to Egyptian pyramids. In its moſt extenſive application, medical arithmetick may be termed what trigonometry, geometry, and the teleſcope are to the arithmetician and aſtronomer, or the compaſs and quadrant to the navigator. By means of it, the higheſt and infinitely the moſt uſeful branches of medicine, the active and practical, may be rendered as certain as any other branches whatſoever of

philoſophy

philoſophy or ſcience. This proſecuted throughout Europe, and the combined information contraſted, aſſimilated, and harmonized, ſeems alone to be wanting, to emancipate our profeſſion from metaphyſical infatuation, and the ſneers of conjecture. There would be no difficulty to prove, that the analytical, metaphyſical, and extemporaneous ſyſtems, from Hippocrates to the eighteenth century, are all defective and erroneous in the plan, materials, foundation, and fabrick. In the figurative ſtile of compariſon, we muſt however confeſs, that the bricklayers have infinitely ſurpaſſed the architects.

AN

ANALYSIS

OF

DISEASES AND MORTALITY.

CHAP. I.

FROM the compound motions of the earth, and of the moon; from the external elements with which the earth and the human ſpecies are inveſted; from their different habitations on the earth; from their different ages; from their different original temperaments, claſs, or genus; from their different ranks and habits of life; from their habitations in city or in country; from the difference of the ſexes, and their ſeparation or intercourſe, myriads

myriads of diseases and deaths ensue, and are peculiarly attached to these various modifications of mankind. Of each of these we are to take a transient glance in the present chapter, as also of the aggregate number of the human species. They are bungling empiricks or audacious prostitutes in medical criticism, who misrepresent the above as speculative and useless propositions in medicine, and who cannot discern the practical tendency of this Introductory Analysis of the Human Species.

A morbid history of the inhabitants of the earth is interwoven with the rudiments of astronomy, geography, and natural philosophy. Our planet is a small link, member, or key of one universal and harmonious system. The vault of Heaven is studded with a profusion of those brilliant orbs; of the sun, and its seven planets, with ten or more of the latter's subordinate satellites, or moons; and of 21 comets. Our ultimate views are lost in the remote and boundless distances of the fixed stars, amounting to some thousands, or perhaps, with their revolving planets, to some millions.

One of the seven planets in our solar system, the earth, this small domain of restless mortals, is distant from the sun 95,000,000 miles. It has several incessant and compound motions. In the space of 365¼ days it completes its annual circle round the sun, which is the length of our year; and throughout that orbit is whirled with the amazing rapidity of 68,000 miles hourly; whereas the swiftness of a cannon ball, in the same interval, is only 480 miles. Its diurnal rotation every 24 hours, like a suspended wheel upon its axis, is, at the equator, at the rate of 1035 miles hourly. Its two remaining motions are the alternate ſpiral inclination and declination of its north and ſouth poles, to and from the ſun at different periods of the year; and the ſmall monthly circle round the common centre of gravity with the moon. From theſe combined terreſtrial motions enſue day and night, ſummer and winter, the equinoxes and ſolſtices. The earth is attended by an inferior, and not very diſtant ſatellite, the moon, its reflecting lamp of night, whoſe influence on the ocean and tides, and in ſome diſeaſes, are univerſally conſpicuous. The ancient aſtrological ſyſtems ſeem to be derived from influences too remote and faint.

Our planet and its inhabitants are inveſted with a few elements, the great and very univerſal agents both of natural good and evil. Heat and light are derived from one common parent, the ſun: their negative qualities, diminution or privation are cold and darkneſs. From the equator to the poles are all the gradations of heat and cold, the extremes of which are ſometimes conſiderably above the human temperature, or 97 of Fahrenheit's thermometer, and ſometimes ſunk conſiderably below 1 or 0 of the ſame ſcale. In both theſe inſtances, as alſo in duration, recurrence and changes, and independent of latitudes, prodigious variations will reſult from the perpendicular or the oblique direction of the ſolar rays, their duration, abſorption, or retention, from elevations, ſoils, ſituations, ſeaſons, days, and nights. But within the equatorial limits the variations in the thermo-

thermometer and ſeaſons are much leſs conſiderable than without the tropicks.

The earth floats in a ſubtile, elaſtick, and ſonorous fluid, the atmoſphere, or air, with which it is circumfuſed on all ſides to the diſtance of more than 45 miles; from whoſe agitations and currents enſue all the diverſity of winds; and whoſe gravity upon the human body, except in elevated ſituations, and in certain changes of weather, amounts to thirty-two thouſand pounds, as is proved by the air-pump and barometer. Its noxious effects may be traced to many ſource to pollution, ſtagnation, unelaſticity, levity, nocturnal chill; the points from whence winds blow, their conſtancy, irregularity, recurrence, velocity.—Another ſubtile, and active agent in the machinery of nature is the electrical emanation; the fabulous artillery and thunder-bolts of Omnipotence.

From the ſun's heat, and the ſucceſſive ſtreams of air and winds, a prodigious evaporation is carried on from the ſurface of the earth, the ocean, and vegetables. This accumulated vapour, to which, according to ſome, the air alſo contributes, is collected into miſts and clouds, and ſuſpended in the atmoſphere, at no great diſtance from the earth, is again diſcharged into the terreſtrial ciſtern in moiſture, fluid or condenſed, as rain, ſnow, hail, but in quantity, duration, recurrence, extent, and contamination, diverſified by a number of collateral cauſes.

Without the concurrent ſupport of theſe different elements, animal and vegetable life would ſoon be annihilated. From each of their ſimple depravities, morbid modifications, defect, or excess, but infinitely more from their complex combinations, intermixtures, and undue assimilations are engendered, and inflict a multitude of human diseases.

In shape the earth has more resemblance to a turnip than to a globe. Its circumference is 24,840 English miles. Its surface is composed of dry land and of water, of which the ocean, without including lakes and rivers, occupies more than double the extent of the land. The dry land is diversified by plains and elevations, none of which ascend to five perpendicular miles.

The Creator has bountifully stored the earth and the ocean with animals and vegetables. Our attention is here circumscribed to the most exalted class, the Human Species; leaving to the naturalist a description of quadrupeds, birds, fishes, insects, and vegetables. By far the largest proportion of the human species are stationed to the north side of the equator, and even to the north of the tropick of cancer. The populous continents, or rather the one vast united continent, of Europe and Asia, and the adjacent islands, comprehending most of the powerful kingdoms in our planet, are in the northern hemisphere. Within the tropical circles and furnace of the earth, are stationed the next considerable hive of mankind. To the south of Capricorn there are few inhabitants. An immense orbicular segment of this hemisphere furnishes habitation for fishes only. But, in the opposite hemisphere, some wretched human beings are scattered through dreary wastes

of

of ice and ſnow within the northern polar circles.

Calculators differ enormouſly reſpecting the *number of the Human Species.* Some ſink the collected herd ſo low as three hundred million, whilſt others exaggerate them to treble and quadruple that amount. It forms no part of my ſcheme to inveſtigate the comparative population of the earth, one, two, and three thouſand years ago. Europe, in all probability, ſince the era of Roman grandeur, has, together with advancement in civilization, likewiſe added to the number of its inhabitants. Thoſe parental nurſeries of the arts and ſciences in Aſia and Africa, have no doubt undergone various revolutions in population. If we were to draw any inferences from the numerous Aſiatic armies, during the ſucceſſive deſpotiſm of Aſſyrian, Babylonian, Medean, and Perſian monarchies, we ſhould conclude that, in remote ages, the ſouth of Aſia abounded in men. The extenſive empire of China, at this day, reſembles an induſtrious bee-hive, and is gorged with mankind. We have ſtill more averſion to plunge into the myſterious archives of Africa, and with critical affectation to pronounce upon the population of that quarter before the decay of its political, commercial, and literary fame with Thebes, Carthage, and Alexandria. That modern-diſcovered tranſatlantic continent, from the cruelties and deſolation of its firſt conquerors, and of a loathſome, infectious diſeaſe exchanged for another, has probably ſuffered conſiderable diminution of its original feeble hive, notwithſtanding the recruit from Europe;

and in the ſcale of population America as yet aſcends to a very ſubordinate rank amongſt the other continents.

The moſt probable calculations eſtimate the whole human race at eight hundred million; of which number Europe, the moſt diminutive in ſize, can boaſt of a hundred and thirty million. The great ſwarm is in Aſia, amounting to between four and five hundred million. Africa is ſuppoſed to contain one third or fourth of the latter number. Over the fertile wilderneſs of America, which ſtands dignified in ſuperior magnitude, are ſcattered not altogether twenty million. On the other hand, in vegetable production Europe is the leaſt prolifick.

But if in London alone, where regiſters of various kinds may be conſulted, calculators are, notwithſtanding, at variance reſpecting its population upwards of one hundred thouſand, and in the whole iſland more than a million; it may be reaſonably ſuſpected, that in forming a groſs eſtimate of the aggregate terreſtrial inhabitants, we may err perhaps one, two, or even three hundred million. As well might we expect a correct liſt of the lions, crocodiles, and monkies of Africa, as of the outcaſt human race in thoſe burning and illiterate regions.

To determine the amount of inhabitants in any city, town, or kingdom, calculators from choice, and oftener from neceſſity, have adopted ſeveral methods. The firſt, and moſt unerring, by a numerical ſurvey through every houſe. The ſecond, by the number of houſes, and by allotting 5 or $4\frac{1}{2}$ inhabitants to each houſe, which, at a general average, including town and country, was found to be the standard in many parts of Europe. But unfortunately in ours, and in many other national registers of houses and separate dwellings, there is great inaccuracy; and in some European cities the inhabitants are double and treble beyond this proportion: The third and far the most fallacious method, both on account of the necessary data, and process, is by multiplying the usual decrement of life, or expectation of an infant at birth in that city or country, whose population we wish to ascertain, by the general medium of christenings.

The assemblages of the human race are greatly diversified by their ages. Dr. Price supposes nearly an equal proportion are living under 16, and above that age; but however, that the latter are most numerous. Davenant states 20 as the partianal number. Dr. Halley supposed the number living under 16 to comprise about one third; and those between 20 and 42 another third of the community. The following table is founded upon a numerical analysis of the inhabitants merely of England, by Davenant. Our table embraces the whole inhabitants of Europe, stating them here at 132,000,000. Each division or group is in the proportion of 13 to 1 more than the inhabitants of the same age in Britain and Ireland; and about 1 to 6 fewer than the whole inhabitants of the earth of a similar description. It is easy to adapt them, "ad libitum," to any numerical extent. We shall hereafter see that the females are considerably more numerous than the males; and that majority is much more conspicuous in the laſt great diviſion of life, that is, after 20 years of age. In this adult and aged diviſion of life, the predominance both of males and females, as contraſted with thoſe under 20, is alſo more conſpicuous in cities than in the country. It is hereafter obſerved, that between one third and fourth of the whole population of Europe are inhabitants of cities and towns.

A TABLE of the INHABITANTS of EUROPE, claſſed according to their Ages.

Ages.		*Numbers.*	
Under 1 year	—	4,080,000	
5 years	—	19,680,000	
10 years	—	36,000,000	
Total under 16 years	—	53,760,000	132,000,000
Total from 16 years to the extreme of exiſtence		78,240,000	
The proportion beyond 60 years		14,200,000	
Of theſe laſt the males		6,280,000	
The females		7,920,000	

It appears from this Table, that the living under 1 year, are four million; between 1 and 5 years, 15 million; between 5 and 10 years, 17 million; between 10 and 20 years, 29 million. That is in all, under 20 years 66 million, or about one half of the inhabitants. Between 20 and 60 years, there are 50 million; from 60 to 100 years and upwards, 14 million.

Extending our views over the ſurface of the globe, we perceive ſtriking diſtinctions between the human ſpecies; not only in the four great Continents, but alſo in different parts of the ſame continent. Theſe differences are principally manifeſt in the colour of the ſkin; in the complexion, countenance, phyſiognomy, hair, form and ſtature. We attend here merely to corporeal diſtinction, without including the intellectual. Theſe great claſſes of mankind may be divided into the European, the Laplander, the Tartar, the Chineſe, the African-negro, and the native American. The modern-diſcovered inhabitants in the iſlands of the Pacific ocean, ſeem to have no remarkable caſt of countenance or figure to ſever them into a ſeparate claſs. Mankind, excluſive of their original mould, as iſſued from the mint of the Creator, are afterwards not only diverſified by climate, ſoil, diet, government, religion, aſſociation, occupation, habit; but throughout a conſiderable extent of the globe, from conqueſt, emigration, colonization, and commercial intercourſe, many nations are now blended and aſſimilated into one; and the elementary characteriſtic features of the aborigines, whether corporeal or mental, more faintly imprinted. Beſides, every one's experience and obſervation will inſtruct him, that in populous kingdoms theſe claſſes branch out into innumerable intermixtures, orders, and genera; and that the ſpecies and varieties are as numerous as the individuals of the human race.

It is of eſſential importance, not only in an enlarged political, but alſo in a medicinal light, to contemplate the various conſtituent portions of human communities; to analyſe the different members and pieces of theſe animated political ſtructures. In a ſtate of nature there are few gradations in ſociety; few profeſſions, or mechanical arts. But by civilization, mankind are

arranged

arranged and connected into an infinite ſeries of deſcending and dependent links. Mr. Voltaire makes only two great diviſions of civilized mankind; the oppreſſors, and the oppreſſed. Deſcending the mole-hill and ladder from the throne to the cottage, we may trace a multitude of gradations in the ſcale of poliſhed communities. We deſcend through nobility and gentry of independent fortunes, in lands or money; through literary profeſſions, including divinity, medicine, law, and various other branches of practical or ſpeculative ſcience; all of which united conſtitute, even in the moſt opulent nations, but a ſmall portion of the community. We next deſcend to a fertile hive of huſbandmen and artizans, laborious drudges in mechanical trades, arts, manufactories, and commerce: to a numerous claſs of retailers or venders of merchandize, and of the neceſſaries of life: to apprentices and clerks throughout the various arts and profeſſions: to ſoldiers, ſailors, domeſtick ſervants: to no inconſiderable multitude buried under ground, and occupied in digging metals and fuel from the bowels of the earth: to infirm, cripples, diſeaſed, puerperal, aged; and to many other links and gradations, which muſt be prodigiouſly diverſified by the variety in governments, religion, climate, national genius, induſtry, commerce, and other cauſes which will occur to philoſophers, and to gentlemen of reflection. They will alſo trace a multitude of diſeaſes not only to theſe ranks, diſtinctions, and employments, but alſo to the active or ſedentary nature of the different profeſſions and arts.

The inhabitants crowded into cities and towns, and thoſe diſperſed in ſmall villages, and in the country, conſtitute other large groups of ſociety. If the reſult of Suſmilch's reſearches and materials, collected throughout Germany, can be depended upon as a criterion for other European nations, the inhabitants in the country are to thoſe in cities and towns as $3\frac{1}{2}$ to 1. Great cities, if we except Rome and Conſtantinople, are of modern date in moſt kingdoms of Europe. In the ninth century, a few towns had been built in Germany; but in England, corporations and conſiderable towns are poſterior to the Norman invaſion. In both ancient and modern times neceſſity alone would naturally collect numbers into thoſe rendezvouſes of ſecurity and defence. Cities, aſſociated communities, and towns, during the religious frenzy of cruſading, and after the termination of this epidemical diſtemper, were aſylums from ariſtocratic tyranny; and when of moderate ſize, are ſeats of politeneſs, refinement, emulation, arts, and ſociety: but when overgrown, they check population; they are drains of the human ſpecies, the graves of infants, and nurſeries of vices. Unfortunately alſo for ſucceeding generations, numerous cities, towns, and harbours, have been founded upon low, unhealthy ſituations, ſurrounded by moraſſes and hills. Moſt cities ſeem to have grown to maturity by accident and time: their ſtreets are narrow, irregular, not ſufficiently ventilated; and the inhabitants abſurdly and pernicioully thronged together. There are moderate-ſized towns, and even country diſtricts, whoſe ſituations are ſo noxious,

noxious, as to make the burials exceed the births: for proofs of which, we need not travel to new uncultivated continents and iſlands, nor to rank tropical climates. In the regular conſtruction and economy of their reſpective cities, vain man is far ſurpaſſed by bees.

Two large and important Claſſes are formed in ſociety, by the diſtinction of the Sexes into male and female. So ſoon as the organs of generation are completely evolved; that is, when the two ſexes arrive at puberty, they are inflamed with a new paſſion and pleaſing ſenſe. In moſt warm climates, this generative period is ſomewhat earlier than in northern latitudes; and in the former alſo, women are ſaid to be more prolifick. We ſhall therefore devote a few words to the union of the ſexes, from whence enſue procreation and births. We cannot poſſibly form any correct judgment of the waſte and expenditure of mankind by diſeaſes and caſualties, without a comparative ſtatement of the recruit. This is an obvious medical, political, and commercial axiom.

The mean ages at which marriages in this iſland commence, is computed from 32 to 35 on the ſide of the man, and 25 on that of the woman: but in this eſtimate ſecond and third marriages are included. Some calculators have computed, that amongſt five million and an half of inhabitants in England, there are annually about forty-one thouſand legal marriages: of which one ſixth part are widows or widowers; about one marriage to every one hundred and four inhabitants; and the annual marriages to the births, as 1 to 4, or $4\frac{1}{2}$.

In cities, not only fewer enter into the matrimonial ſtate, but the product alſo of city and country marriages is obſerved to differ. Marriages in cities, one with another, ſeldom produce above four; generally between three and four, and ſometimes not three children: whereas country and village marriages ſeldom produce leſs than four, and generally between four and five at a medium; for ſome married pairs have only one or two; others ſix, eight, twelve, or more; and a ſmall remnant are unprolifick. Whether this diſparity between the product of city and country marriages is to be imputed to diſſipation, libertiniſm, and incontinence, both in the ſingle and married ſtate; to the cloudy apprehenſions and fears of overſtocking their houſe; to later, fewer, and leſs frequent unions in the matrimonial bond; or to all theſe and other cauſes combined, I ſubmit to the reader's conſideration.

Natural, or illegitimate children, are enrolled in the public records of chriſtenings, and ſwell their proportion to the regiſtered weddings ſomewhat greater than they would appear without this extraneous addition. In ſome German regiſters, Dr. Short found, that of 333,655 births, the illegitimate amounted to one thirty-ſeventh part; and in an inland town of England, that of 10,337 births, 284, or about one thirtieth part, were illegitimate.

Providence has wiſely ordained, that throughout thoſe European kingdoms, of which we have any regiſters, a few more males ſhould be born

born than females; and indeed ſuch a ſurplus is rendered neceſſary from the waſte by wars, emigration, intemperance, mechanical arts and trades, the inclemency and viciſſitudes of the weather and ſeaſons, the vices and misfortunes to which political puniſhments are annexed, with various other noxious caſualties, to all which the male ſex are moſt expoſed. In Dr. Arbuthnot's Table, printed in the London Philoſophical Tranſactions, of the proportion between the births of the ſexes, in 46 years were baptized, of males 329,742; of females 308,644; majority of males only 23,098. By the London regiſters, from 1657 to 1776, I find that there have been chriſtened of males, 1,041,149; of females, 983,061; or as 18 to 17: and therefore, that in this long interval of 120 years, and comprehending two million of births, there is only a trifling majority of males, amounting to 58,088; a number which would ſcarce recruit the conſumption of a few active campaigns. In volume the 7th of the Philoſophical Tranſactions abridged, there is an account of the annual births during ſeveral years at Vienna, Breſlaw, Dreſden, Leipſick, and Ratiſbon; and in thoſe cities male and female births were as 19 to 18. Amongſt the abortives and ſtill-born we alſo find a plurality of males.

If the regiſters can be depended upon, it appears that there are more births in winter than in ſummer, not only in town but alſo in the country. The increaſed population during the winter, in cities, muſt naturally augment the births. But although the fruit of the human womb may not have arrived at maturity before winter,

winter, it is no proof againſt the general law of the ſpring and ſummer influence on animals and vegetables in contributing to fecundity and generation. We muſt diſtinguiſh between the ſpring and harveſt of human fertility.

If the number of inhabitants in any kingdom, city, or village, continues the ſame without increaſe or decreaſe, and ſupported by their own procreation only, it is evident, that there the annual births and burials will be equal, and the ſupply proportioned to the waſte; and in equal numbers, as many will die at all ages as are born in the year, on a general average; and the numbers dying any year at one, two, three years of age, and ſo on to the extreme of exiſtence, will be juſt equal with the numbers who ſucceſſively attain to thoſe different ages at which the others die.

The total annual births amongſt five million and an half of inhabitants in England, are calculated by Davenant at 190,000; which is about one birth to every twenty-five inhabitants; and amongſt ten million of inhabitants in Britain and Ireland, the annual procreation will exceed three hundred and fifty thouſand; and the annual mortality ſhould be ſomewhat inferior. In the kingdom of Pruſſia, from the year 1715 to 18, there were chriſtened, at an annual medium, 78,826; buried, 55,852. In the kingdom of Sweden, the annual average of births during nine years, ending in 1763, was 90,240; burials, 69,125. In Norway, in 1761, the chriſtenings were 11,024; burials, 6,926. In France, during three years, ending in 1772, the annual average of births was 920,918; burials,

rials, 780,040. In the county diſtrict of Vaux, in Switzerland, during ten years, the births were 3,155; burials, 2,504. The country, ſays Graunt, has 6,339 births for 5,280 burials. In that little fertile iſland Madeira, the inhabitants have been computed to double themſelves in eighty-four years; ſo great is the difference between the births and burials. And in ſome provinces of North America, if Dr. Franklin's calculations are correct; the inhabitants double themſelves in the ſhort ſpace of twenty-five, twenty-two, and even fifteen years.

On the other hand, in all the large cities of Europe; in Paris, Vienna, Rome, Dreſden, Berlin, Amſterdam, London, Edinburgh, Dublin, and in almoſt all towns of conſiderable magnitude and population, the total annual births are inferior to the burials. It is calculated, that in London, within the laſt 150 years, near a million more of the human ſpecies have been waſted, beyond what were reared by its own original growth and procreation. But in ſmall villages and country diſtricts, the annual births exceed the burials; and it is from this redundance that a ſupply is furniſhed for the extraordinary conſumption of armies, navies, war, colonization, emigration; excluſive of ſickneſs, and other morbid caſualties: the country and village ſurplus prevents depopulation. There are about 4½ million of births annually in Europe, and the deaths are inferior, probably by half a million. Wars however are here excepted, which will alſo detract from the births.

But

But if, on one hand, large cities and high refinement are obſtacles to population, a wild ſtate of nature is ſtill more detrimental. There are more inhabitants concentrated into one large metropolis of Aſia or Europe, than could be collected in many thouſand miles of the North American wilderneſs on its firſt diſcovery. A medium ſtate between the vicious extremes of refinement and rude ſavageneſs; or the middle ſtages between the iron and golden ages of the ancient philoſophers, is the moſt favourable to the increaſe of our ſpecies. But the cauſes conducive to population and depopulation are of infinite compaſs, and are of a compound nature medical and political. They are connected with the ſtate of government, religion, climate, genius, induſtry, riches, poverty, taxes, luxury, refinement, diſſipation, profligacy, wars, colonization, emigration, commerce, agriculture, the unequal diſtribution and monopoly of property and farms, the plenty, ſcarcity, and cheapneſs of food, the encouragement or diſcouragement of matrimony, and with many other cauſes cloſely allied to our future medical inveſtigation. Once for all, I embrace the preſent opportunity to obſerve, that throughout this treatiſe there are hints and ideas, each of which draws a whole train after them: the full open detail, and ample diſcovery is left to the reader.

CHAP.

CHAP. II.

WE are now to view the human race unexpectedly arrested, and struggling in the tragical and last stages of their terrestrial pilgrimage. The vision of human life is soon at an end: we are ushered into the world with lamentable exclamation; and are too often torn out of it in pain and agony. Bills of Mortality, however defective and inaccurate, yet sufficiently demonstrate this awful truth, that very few of the human species die of old age, or natural decay: by far the greater proportion are prematurely cut off by diseases. Of all the animal tribe, who usually bring forth one at a birth, none perish in such numbers in infancy: almost one half of human mortality is under five years of age. In London, Vienna, Berlin, and every other overgrown metropolis of Europe, on an average, one half of the children born, die under three years of age. But in country towns and villages, the proportion of infant mortality greatly abates. In some country towns of England, of considerable magnitude and population, as Manchester, half the children die under five; at Norwich, half under six; at Northampton, half under ten years of age. London, therefore, will have lost, out of equal capitals, a number in the intermediate space, between three and ten, more than Northampton.

Attend next to the small proportion of Infant Mortality in open country districts. By Dr. Short's

Short's regiſters of ſeveral ſmall country villages in England, the major part born live to the ages of 25, 27, 33, and 40. In many healthy country pariſhes, half the inhabitants born live to 40, 46, and a few even to 50 and 60; and rear large families of children. In ſome extenſive country diſtricts of Switzerland, ſimilar obſervations have been made by Suſmilch and Muret. Here, therefore, is an aſtoniſhing diſparity between the proſpects of city and country life, in the early ſtages of puerile exiſtence. Infants in cities reſemble tender plants excluded from freſh air, or fiſh confined in ſtagnant water; and periſh before they can acquire a ſolidity and ſeaſoning to endure the adulterated quality of the ſurrounding element.

Mortality, univerſally, during the firſt year after birth, is the moſt enormous in the funeral catalogue: it is nearly one fourth of the mortality of Europe. A London infant at birth, has but an equal chance of living to three years old; whereas in the country, as before obſerved, half of thoſe born ſurvive to maturity. Upon reaching the third year, in cities, infants are ſomewhat ſeaſoned, and the hurricane of puerile carnage is greatly abated. There is not afterwards ſuch a prodigious diſproportion between city and country mortality; and, in a few years after, between ſeven and ten, they approach nearer to an equality. Death is earlier glutted with ſlaughter in cities, than in the country. From the London regiſters of burials, it appears that more die in the metropolis under two years of age, than from two to upwards of forty; and more under five years of age, than from five

to

to between fifty and ſixty: yet under five, there are but an inconſiderable number alive, compared to the latter claſs above that age: the deaths are greatly diſproportioned to the living numbers or capitals. A few more die in London in the ſhort interval between five and ten years of age, than in the ſucceeding double interval from ten to twenty; and more between twenty and thirty, than in the fifteen preceding years; and the burial liſt continues turgid to ſixty. Between eight and ſixteen years of age, one of every ſeventy of the Chriſt School boys is computed to die. Davenant rates the decrement in theſe years at only one *per cent.* Having ſurmounted all the dangers and precipices of the early preceding journey, there is no ſtage wherein the future proſpects of exiſtence and longevity are ſo extenſive: during thoſe years of adoleſcence, very few die in city, town, or country. The tide of life is then at the flood; and from thence to the ultimate verge of exiſtence, vitality continues gradually to ebb. Towards the meridian of life, it ſinks to two; and at ſixty down to four or five *per cent.*

One reaſon, but not the only one, as calculators alledge, of the great ſurge in the London bills, from twenty up to forty, is, that within this interval of life, the majority of extraneous new ſettlers or recruits arrive; and conſequently augment the burials in the metropolis, from twenty to forty, beyond their natural proportion: the principal reaſon is, a univerſal law of nature in every ſituation; the cauſes and explanation of which will be found

in

in the hiſtory of diſeaſes. After paſſing the meridian, and in the evening of life, the ſeaſoned inhabitants of cities are ſaid, by Dr. Price, to have the advantage of the country, in health and longevity: that is to ſay, although the number who have ſurvived in the country to ſixty, ſeventy, and eighty, are greater proportionally than in cities, yet the latter claſs arrived at thoſe years in London have, comparatively, ſurer expectations of life. I do not, however, find this aſſertion verified in fact; the balance, if any, vibrating alternately on each ſide. Nearly one fifth of the annual mortality, promiſcuouſly, is after 60 years of age; and about one half of theſe, or one tenth or twelfth of the whole, are left to moulder by the irremediable dilapidations of time. The proportion of inhabitants who reach eighty years of age are computed, in London and Vienna, at one of every forty: but in country pariſhes, at one of every twenty-two; and in ſome, even one of every eleven. In both city and country, the few ſurvivors at ninety, out of each thouſand coetaneous births, will have loſt almoſt all their fellow-travellers in the journey, long before reaching that goal; and about three or four only out of each thouſand, on an average, will be then left alive.

There are indeed a few inſtances of extraordinary Longevity, to 150 and 165; ſuch are Jenkins and Par, in this iſland. In Bacon Lord Verulam's Hiſtory of Long Livers, male and female; their climate, diet, mode of life, appetites, exerciſes, ſtudies, paſſions, diſpoſitions, habits, and complexions, were exceedingly

ingly diſſimilar. It is however probable, from obſervation and analogy, that the indigent and laborious claſs of mankind do not attain to longevity in the ſame proportion with the middling and more opulent ranks. The wandering Savages of America are notoriouſly ſhort-lived. Throughout Europe, Aſia, Africa, and America, the rich, the poor, the inhabitants of city and country, with very different complexion, climate, ſoil, diet, and conveniences, all ſeldom exceed the uſual term of life allotted to man: ſeventy and eighty is mentioned in holy writ, as the brink of our earthly duration. Since the days of Moſes; that is, between three and four thouſand years, human exiſtence has been circumſcribed within the ſame narrow bounds. In the London regiſters of mortality, during a period of thirty years, from 1728 to 1758, the total mortality is 750,332; and of all this number, 242 only reached beyond 100 years of age; one cf whom arrived at 138. Throughout the annual mortality of Europe, which we have eſtimated at four million, there are not probably two thouſand who have compleated a century; nor throughout the globe twelve thouſand of this deſcription.

In ſome races and families of men, longevity ſeems to be hereditary; and his age, though little more than a dream, exceeds that of all other living creatures, a few only excepted. Amongſt the quadruped creation, the elephant ſurpaſſes man in longevity: amongſt the birds, the Swan, and a few others, have ſurvived upwards of a century. The age of fiſhes is determined with more ingenuity than certainty: ſome ſeem to rival man in years. But among the numerous vegetable tribes, the oak, cheſtnut, and ſome other lords of the foreſt, ſurvive centuries.

On contraſting the mortality of Males and Females, it appears, that, notwithſtanding the ſurplus of male births, the perils of child-bearing, the many vexatious diſeaſes peculiar to the fair ſex, and that phyſicians and apothecaries have many more patients of the latter; yet the total aggregate number of living females exceeds that of males, in moſt European kingdoms. Upon a numerical inqueſt in Edinburgh, and ſome other great cities, it was found, that females were to males as 4 to 3: in London, as 13 to 10; and in ſome other cities and towns, as 9 to 8. But in country diſtricts, Graunt and Suſmilch agree, that the two ſexes approach nearer to an equality. In the province of Jerſey, in North America, the males were found the majority. From 1702 to 1752; that is, during a period of fifty years, I find the proportion of male and female mortality in London as follows: Male deaths, 618,076; Female deaths, 626,692. Whence, therefore, does it happen, that female deaths preponderate over the male, when more of the latter are born, and, as calculators aſſert, the mortality of males, at all ages, is greater than that of females? As a ſolution of this difficulty and partial exception, I ſhould ſuggeſt a greater exportation and tranſportation of males to the ſea and land ſervice, to nautical commerce, and to unhealthy climates.

Even in the marriage ſtate, the chance of ſurvivorſhip ſeems conſiderably in favour of the

wife.

wife. In Breslaw, during eight years, five married men died to three married women. Susmilch, on a scrutiny through several kingdoms and principalities of Germany, found, that three married men died to two married women. Dr. Price estimates the chance in favour of the wife being the survivor in marriage, as 3 to 2; and this calculation is confirmed by the experience of the general Clerical Society in Scotland, who have long established funds to support their widows. From their records, it appears that twenty married clergymen have died to twelve wives; or, as 5 to 3. By an accurate survey of several principalities and cities in Germany, and collected by Susmilch, the widows were to the widowers as 3, and even 4 to 1. At marriage, it should be observed, there is generally a disparity of age; the bridegroom is from six to twelve years older than the bride; and therefore should, in the course of nature, die sooner: and perhaps also more widowers, comparatively with the other sex, enter into a second marriage; which tends to reduce their numbers. Besides, husbands are more exposed to the vicissitudes of the weather and seasons, to excessive labour, and noxious trades, and to many other causes of diseases.

Dr. Price finds, that the sexes respectively commence to be widowers and widows about 52 and 44; that is, men and women entering into matrimony, on a general average, at the ages of 33 and 25, will become widowers and widows at 52 and 44: consequently, that each marriage will be dissolved by the death of one of them, in nineteen years; which is the ultimate term and probability of the husband and wife being both alive. For although some marriages may be protracted forty and fifty years, yet others may be dissolved in one year, or in a shorter time.

We have not yet sufficient information to determine the comparative chances of Female Longevity in the married and single state. At Berlin, indeed, calculators have remarked, that there were more married women alive at great ages, than of those who remained single. But such result might naturally be expected from a greater proportion in the decline of life of widows and wives, compared to antiquated virgins. From the ages of fifteen to twenty-five, married women likewise are said to have the advantage of the single, in whom the dictates of nature are frustrated and violated.

Comparing the mortality of the Seasons, Dr. Short found, from a variety of country registers, that mortality general begins its reign in December; that at March it is in its zenith; and at May in its declension. In twenty-five country towns and parishes, he found the winter to the summer mortality as 50 to 41. At Manchester, a country town of England, Dr. Percival found the winter to the summer mortality as 11 to 8. At Vevey in Switzerland, during sixty years, Mr. Muret found the burials, during the four winter months, as 5 to 4 to those of the summer. Another proof of this is recorded in the *Recherches sur la Population, par Messance:* The total sick admitted into the *Hotel Dieu* hospital in Paris, from 1724 to 1763 (forty years) were, in the four winter months, December,

January,

January, February, and March, 314,824; and in the four ſummer months, June, July, Auguſt, September, 238,522; or as 4 to 3. In London too, the undertaker's harveſt is in winter. There is one obvious reaſon why, in every metropolis, the winter mortality ſhould exceed that of ſummer, from the greater concourſe of inhabitants of all ranks; but independent of additional population in winter, the ſame law ſeems to prevail in country places. Whether from diſeaſes originally engendered in that ſeaſon, or from its more pernicious effects on the lingering and convaleſcent train of chronic and acute diſeaſes, may be diſputed. Within the tropical circles there is not the ſame diverſity of the ſeaſons as in European regions: there the periodical hurricane and rainy ſeaſon, or monſoon, is the moſt ſickly and fatal.

On collating the annual average of deaths, at all ages, in a ſickly year of London, and other great cities, with ſickly years in the country pariſhes, Dr. Short found, that cities and towns have the advantage of the country, and are leſs annoyed. According to this author, in ſpacious open country diſtricts, where fatal epidemick diſtempers burſt out, the burials not only exceeded the chriſtenings, but more died in one year, than during 6, 10, 12, or ſometimes 15 healthy years; whereas he adds, in London, and ſuch other cities, not above one third, fourth, or fifth, beyond the ordinary conſumption, are ſwept away. Peſtilential mortality alone is the ſolitary exception to the Doctor's propoſition. In the London morbid regiſters we may frequently obſerve, that in different months the deaths are double or treble above equal periods of the ſame year: but during the preſent century, I find no inſtance even of triple, and very rarely of double exceſs, in the annual London burials. Dr. Short adds, that mortality is more regular and conſtant in cities, and not ſo many deſtroyed, "per ſaltum," from raging epidemicks, as in the country. In pure open air he ſuggeſts, that contagion and infection, and other adulterated effluvia, are more virulent. Or, perhaps he ſhould have ſaid, at leaſt have added, that in cities where the atmoſphere is charged with a load of ſmoke, and other heterogeneous vapours, epidemical poiſons may be blunted, decompounded, or annihilated: that likewiſe in cities human bodies are more early ſeaſoned and habituated to ſuch noxious impreſſions, and like doctors and nurſes, are in ſome degree fortified by habit: that beſides in every large metropolis, ſmall-pox, meaſles, nervous, putrid, and ſome other febrile epidemicks, are almoſt conſtant reſidents; and conſequently the devaſtation from theſe diſeaſes is more regular and equal than in the country, where there are ſeveral years and more irregular diſtances between their invaſions.

Let us condenſe our calculations into a few general abſtracts of human carnage. If we ſcan the manſions of diſeaſe and woe, we find, on an average, 1 death, annually, out of every 5 families in cities: but in country towns, and open diſtricts, 1 out of 7, 8, 9; and in a few healthy places, 1 out of every 10 families. Including the whole aſſemblage of inhabitants in city, town, and country, from birth to the extreme

of

of exiſtence, they are computed to die in the following annual proportion to the living: In London, 1 of 21; Dublin, 1 of 22; Edinburgh, 1 of 21; Vienna, 1 of 20; Amſterdam, 1 of 22; Berlin, 1 of 26; but, diſmal to relate, of the oppreſſed negroes in the Weſt India iſlands, 1 of 7. This is nearly Dr. Price's calculation; but Halley and Suſmilch compute only 1 of 22 to 29 to die annually in cities. In ſmaller cities and towns, ſuch as Norwich and Northampton, the general average of deaths is 1 of 24 to 26; but in ſeveral provinces and healthy country villages, 1 of 32 and 33, up to 45, 50, and even 60, is the annual drain: 1 of 43 to 50 was the average in upwards of a thouſand country pariſhes on the continent; and recorded in Suſmilch. Within the above ſhort intervals of time, there will have died in the reſpective cities and country places enumerated, a number equal to the whole inhabitants.

The ancient Egyptians computed a century by 3 generations; thus eſtabliſhing an auxiliary regulator of chronology and hiſtory. At this day 33 or 35 is near the meaſure of a generation, and the general decreaſe of a community throughout Europe, comprehending all the inhabitants in city, village, and country: that is, mankind ſhare amongſt them from about 32 or 33 to 35 years each of exiſtence: and within this fugitive interval of time, a number equal to all the preſent inhabitants of this iſland, or of the whole earth, will be exterminated. If we extend this eſtimate to the whole human race, eight hundred million will die in 33 years; twenty-four million annually; ſeventy thouſand daily; three

 thouſand

thousand hourly; and fifty every minute. It is perhaps superfluous to add, that, in the same intervals, an equal or superior number will be born.

According to De Moivre and Dr. Price, "the probabilities or expectation of life, decrease as we advance from childhood to old age, in an arithmetical progression; that is, in such a manner that the difference is always the same between the number of persons living at the beginning of any one year, and the number living at the beginning of the following year." Or, in other words, less enveloped in mathematical obscurity, out of any specified number, an hundred or a thousand, the same proportion will continue to die every year until near 80 years of age and upwards: consequently, the probabilities of life are constantly decreasing; because notwithstanding the progressive annual drain from the capitals, yet the deaths continue throughout equal. But this proportion is certainly erroneous in the first stages of life, and until about 10.

View the above proposition in another light. From any given number there will be an equal drain annually, until what De Moivre terms the *complement* or *maximum*, or utmost probable extreme of life, which he fixes at 86, all are dead. The probability, therefore, that the whole of any limited number whatsoever, or age, will all be exterminated is the number of years between 86 and the year such a number are all alive. Of 56 persons alive at 30, they should all be dead in 56 years, because 56 added to 30 amounts to 86, the maximum: of 46 persons alive at 40 years

years of age, they ſhould all be dead in 46 years: and 36 perſons alive at 50 years of age, ſhould be dead in 36 years; for 50 and 36 complete the maximum. Again, the expectation of any ſingle life is only half the maximum or complement, or half the ſpace between that age and the above ultimate term of exiſtence: but here we muſt repeat the former exception, and draw the line after 10 years of age.

The expectation of *two* equal joint lives, according to De Moivre, is only one third of the complement of life. Example: two lives, aged 40, have an even chance or probable proſpect of continuing together in exiſtence only 15 years; which is the third of the complement, reckoning from 40 to 86: the expectation of the ſurvivor is alſo 15 years. Or, ſuppoſe a lot of marriages of perſons at 40 years of age, they will, on an average, continue together 15½ years; and the ſurvivors the ſame time after. This expectation, therefore, is the probable duration of each marriage, and the ſhare of each perſon's life. But it may be proper to add, that the duration of marriages, and the value of ſingle and joint lives, will, on a promiſcuous calculation, be different from the regiſters of annuitant and inſurance offices; becauſe they are ſcrupulouſly vigilant to exclude all diſeaſed and unhealthy perſons from becoming members.

The following Chart and Tables, preſent a diſtinct proſpect of the fates clipping the mortal thread, from birth to old age, in city and country. But we are not to ſuppoſe that in every inſtance there will be annually a regular arithmetical diminution, as marked in the different tables:

tables: ſome years will be more fatal than others; and we are to form eſtimates from an average of ſeveral years. Throughout the Chart the firſt column points out the age, the ſecond the number living at that age, the third the number who die during the year; and ſo on to the end of each table. But obſerve, that the number of infants, at the beginning of the ſecond column, are ſuppoſed to be all born together on the firſt day of that year; and this rule applies throughout all the remaining ages, From the Chart, and from the ſubſequent different Tables may be eſtimated the annual waſte, out of any ſpecified number, at all ages, the ultimate proſpects of exiſtence, and the odds or probability of a perſon in health ſurviving a ſtated number of years. Theſe are alſo adapted to all ages, and to the inhabitants of city, and country. It would be endleſs to point out the inſtances of their utility and practical application. The two intermediate ſhort Tables demonſtrate both the total amount, and the gradations of annual mortality, at different ages, in London and in Europe.

In one of the ſhort tables juſt now alluded to, I have attempted, as nearly as ſuch an intricate and unprecedented ſubject would permit, or at leaſt as I was enabled from any probably data, to preſent at one view the *annual mortality*, and compa ative decrement, throughout all ages, of the inhabitants of Europe, including city, town, and country. We may, in ſome degree, judge of the mortality, comparatively, by the numbers alive in the different intervals of life; and by an average of city and country mortality in each of thoſe intervals. The annual mortality of Great Britain and Ireland, in each of the following intervals of life, will, in correſpondence with the population, be inferior, as 1 to 13, to that of Europe; and the latter as 1 to 6, to that of all the human ſpecies. (See a Table in the preceding chapter.)

A TABLE of the Annual Mortality in London, from 1728, to 1743, at different Ages, taken at an Annual Medium, by Dr. SHORT.

	Years of Age.			Died.
	Under	——	2	9910
From	2	to	5	2411
	5	——	10	980
	10	——	20	851
	20	——	30	2060
	30	——	40	2471
	40	——	50	2510
	50	——	60	2231
	60	——	70	1675
	70	——	80	1200
	80	——	90	634
	90	——	100	117
Total Annual Medium of Deaths in this Period				27,058

A TABLE

A TABLE of the Annual Mortality throughout Europe, including Cities, Towns, and Country.

Years of age.		Total annual proportion of deaths in those intervals.	Comparative proportion of deaths to the living in those intervals.
Under 1	—	1,000,000	1 of 4, or 25 per cent.
From	1 to 5	800,000	1 of 19, or 5 per cent.
	5 to 10	180,000	1 of 86, or nearly 1 per cent.
	10 to 20	260,000	not altogether 1 per cent.
	20 to 60	900,000	nearly 2 per cent.
	60 to 100 and upwards	860,000	1 of 16, or about 6 per cent.
		4,000,000	

The two following TABLES are taken from Dr. Price. I have however omitted the fractions.

The probable Expectations or Prospects of Life in

Ages.	London.	Vienna.	Berlin.	Country parish of Brandenburg.	Holy Cross, near Shrewsbury.	Pais de Vaud, in Switzerland.
At birth	18 yrs.	17 yrs.	18 yrs.	33 yrs.	33 yrs.	37 yrs.
Age 12	34	36	36	44	44	44
25	26	28	27	36	35	35
30	24	26	25	32	32	31
35	22	23	24	26	28	28
40	20	21	21	25	26	24
45	18	18	19	22	23	21
50	16	16	16	18	20	18
55	14	14	14	15	17	15
60	13	12	13	12	15	12
65	11	10	11	10	12	10
70	9	9	9	8	10	8
75	7	7	7	6	8	6
80	5	6	6	5	5	5

The Odds or Probability of living ONE *Year in*

Ages.	London.	Vienna.	Berlin.	Country parish of Brandenburg.	Holy Cross, near Shrewsbury.	Pais de Vaud, in Switzerland.
At birth	2 to 1	2 to 1	2 to 1	4 to 1	5 to 1	5 to 1
Age 12	75 to 1	84 to 1	123 to 1	112 to 1	144 to 1	160 to 1
25	56 to 1	66 to 1	50 to 1	110 to 1	100 to 1	117 to 1
30	45 to 1	56 to 1	44 to 1	107 to 1	96 to 1	111 to 1
40	31 to 1	36 to 1	32 to 1	78 to 1	55 to 1	83 to 1
50	24 to 1	27 to 1	30 to 1	50 to 1	50 to 1	49 to 1
60	18 to 1	19 to 1	18 to 1	25 to 1	26 to 1	23 to 1
70	12 to 1	11 to 1	12 to 1	11 to 1	16 to 1	10 to 1
80	7 to 1	7 to 1	7 to 1	6 to 1	8 to 1	4 to 1

CHAP. III.

HAVING in the preceding Chapter endeavoured to eſtabliſh the mortality of the human ſpecies at different ages, I am now to attempt a more arduous taſk; to aſcertain the mortality by different diſeaſes and caſualties. I propoſe therefore, in imitation of the geographers, to ſpread out and to review, in one general Chart, the enormous hoſt of diſeaſes which diſgorge their virulence over the earth, and, with frightful rapacity, wage inceſſant hoſtilities with mankind. By this means, we ſhall, to uſe a military phraſe, reconnoitre more diſtinctly our

our enemies arranged in hoſtile front; and be warned to make the beſt diſpoſition and preparation for defence where the greateſt danger is apprehended, and the moſt formidable aſſaults to be ſuſtained. Armed with diſeaſes, the grim King of Terrors appears in the moſt hideous aſpect. Under all theſe predatory diſguiſes and morbifick forms, I ſhall track him grappling with mankind, and with his tremendous ſcythe mowing down generations.

I could eaſily have exhibited tables of the Diſeaſes and Caſualties in London during the greater part of the laſt century. But, compared to its preſent magnitude, the Britiſh metropolis was then inſignificant in ſize: 23 new pariſhes have been ſince gradually added to the London bills: there is alſo a chaſm in that century of 10 years in which the regiſters are loſt. Again, until 1665 and 6, London was infeſted with the plague; which diſeaſe, previous to that date, ſeems to have been one primary object of the regiſters: and to adopt Graunt and Short's ſentiments, theſe records, from various political and religious obſtacles, were then very negligently managed. During the early part of this interval, the kingdom was diſtracted with civil war; and after the great peſtilence in 1665, London muſt have required ſome years to recruit. Beſides, had I attempted to form tables for even the latter part of the laſt century, the reader would have been fruitleſſly embarraſſed; and ſuch an attempt muſt ever prove abortive. For example, under one and the ſame title, in the annually bills of mortality, are often confounded flox, ſmall pox, and meaſles: conſumptions and tiſſick: cancer, canker, and thruſh: wolf, cancer, gangrene, and fiſtula: cancer, gangrene, fiſtula, and mortification: gout and ſciatica: vapours and water in the head: quinſey and thruſh: teeth and worms: ſores, ulcers, bruiſed and broken limbs: cough, cold, and chincough, &c. Theſe are a few ſpecimens of Noſological abſurdity in the ſuperintendants of the public regiſters.

Notwithſtanding this rabble of diſeaſes, in commenting upon the London bills and diſeaſes of the preſent century, I conſtantly refer back, and contraſt them with the bills of the laſt thirty years of the preceding century; ſo that, as near as the imperfection of the materials will admit, the mortality and diſeaſes of 105 years in London is preſented at one view; and comprehends the various acute and chronic diſeaſes, by which about two million and a half of the human ſpecies have been deſtroyed. The few authors who have written on bills of mortality, have obſcured their works in a cloud of figures and calculation: the reader muſt have no ſmall portion of phlegm and reſolution to follow them throughout with attention: they often tax the memory and patience with a numerical ſuperfluity, even to a nuiſance.

For the above and many other reaſons, I have compreſſed into one chart, the London Diſeaſes and Caſualties of ſeventy-five years in the preſent century: each diſeaſe and caſualty is arranged in a progreſſive ſeries of fifteen years mortality; and in a fifth column is added together the mortality of the preceding five diviſions. During this period, London has been more

more populous and ſtationary in numbers: and by this means, the actual and comparative magnitude, riſe, and declenſion of different diſeaſes, will be more conſpicuous in each period or interval: and by meaſuring the mortality with the population, we are enabled, with certain precautions and exceptions, to make the diſeaſes and caſualties of London ſerve as a morbid barometer to the whole nation, and in ſome degree to the whole univerſe.

The important reaſon which determined me in forming an arrangement of fifteen years, in preference to any other number or period, was, that the annual havock by ſimilar diſeaſes and caſualties, throughout this and the neighbouring iſland, might be computed with ſome probability by each fifteen years of the London bills; and thereby to elicite a new, curious, and comprehenſive propoſition in medicine. For inſtance, if we ſuppoſe the ſtanding number, on an average, of the London inhabitants at ſeven hundred thouſand; and the total inhabitants in Britain and Ireland at ten million; and if the ſame diſeaſes and caſualties were equally diffuſed and fatal to this whole community, then, in ſuch caſe, the London bills and our chart would ſerve as a ſcale or index of mortality to both kingdoms: as many would die annually of every diſeaſe and caſualty throughout ten million, as are cut off in fifteen years in London; for ſeven hundred thouſand multiplied by fifteen, amounts nearly to ten million. The exceſs is trifling in a general calculation upon ſo large a ſcale.

But to ſupply the probable deficiency in the annual mortality of London by different diſeaſes

and

and caſualties, we muſt make an addition to each of one fourth. To the mortality of ſmall-pox, in London, during fifteen years, and rated at thirty thouſand, we ſhould add one fourth more to raiſe it to its juſt ſtandard; that is, to about thirty-eight thouſand; which would be the annual mortality amongſt ten million in Britain and Ireland, ſuppoſing ſmall-pox equally univerſal, one time or other, and deſtructive. By the ſame hypotheſis, amongſt one hundred and thirty million in Europe Variolous mortality annually, would amount to upwards of four hundred thouſand; and, amongſt eight hundred million, that is the whole human race, to nearly two million and a half annually.

Let us view on this great ſcale the annual havock of a few diſeaſes, aſſuming London as a radix to Britain and Ireland, and the latter to Europe. It appears, that the *annual devaſtation* from fevers remittent, nervous, and putrid, and their ſpecies, in Britain and Ireland, is 60,000; throughout Europe, 800,000; from ſmall pox in Britain and Ireland, 38,000; throughout Europe, 494,000: meaſles are only one tenth of ſmall-pox: conſumptions, at leaſt in this iſland, are ſtill more deleterious than fevers: from aſthma and dyſpnea, in Britain and Ireland, upwards of 10,000; throughout Europe upwards of 100,000: apoplexy is inferior by one half to aſthma: from dropſy, in Britain and Ireland, 17,000; throughout Europe, 170,000: from child-bed, in Britain and Ireland, 4000; throughout Europe, 50,000: from dead births, or abortions, at or near maturity, in Britain and Ireland, 13,000; throughout Europe, 130,000:

aged, in Britain and Ireland, 31,000; throughout Europe, 400,000; that is, according to our preceding Table in the former Chapter of the annual mortality of Europe, nearly one half of those deaths beyond 60 years of age. The annual mortality throughout the universe will be in the ratio of 6 to 1 beyond Europe.

On the above simple principle, a sort of medical trigonometry and geometry, a gross estimate may be formed of the annual havock throughout mankind, by every other disease and casualty, taking the precaution, however, to attend to the subsequent criticisms on the London bills, and on diseases in general. From these Tables and Commentaries we are also furnished with a key to the comparative mortality of each disease amongst a community, and its devastation numerically.

Another very curious and useful corollary may be grounded on the above hypothesis; which is, from the proportion of deaths, to form a probable conjecture of the numbers who are annually sick, or afflicted with different diseases in a community. Example: if one of every seven die of the small-pox, and the variolous deaths throughout Britain and Ireland are rated at 38,000 annually, this number, multiplied by seven, amounts to 266,000 annually infected in both Islands with variolous contagion. Apply the same rule to childbed mortality; rate the annual havock by parturition in the two islands at 4,000: it will hereafter be shewn, that in London one of seventy-four women die in childbed: multiply therefore 4,000 by 74, the product is 296,000, which is not very distant, although inferior to the total annual procreation in both iſlands. And in theſe two examples, I have ſuggeſted what may be termed an inverſe proof of both propoſitions. Upon the ſame principles a groſs eſtimate may be formed of the numbers afflicted with dropſy, and with many other diſeaſes.

Gentlemen who have not particularly attended to the ſubject of morbid calculations (and very few of the medical profeſſion have) will, on better information, be aſtoniſhed at the flagrant errors daily committed by authors when treating of theſe topicks. Out of the many examples which might be enumerated, I ſhall merely ſelect one in proof. Baron Dimſdale, in a Treatiſe on Inoculation, dedicated to the preſent Empreſs of Ruſſia, calculated that, at leaſt, two million were annually deſtroyed by ſmall-pox alone in the Ruſſian empire; and it was not until after the publication of my Obſervations on his different Inoculating Eſſays, that this error and others were eraſed.

I would requeſt the reader's particular attention to another circumſtance: which is, that on comparing the gradations of mortality in the following chart, we are not to eſtimate the relative number, frequency, or proportion of certain diſeaſes, compared to others by the abſolute mortality of each. For inſtance, Apoplexy kills rather more annually in London than meaſles; but yet the latter diſeaſe is infinitely more univerſal and diffuſed amongſt the community, and conſequently leſs dangerous to life: cancerous and venereal caſes are widely different in the annual number afflicted with each, although the deaths are not far diſtant from an equality. The ſame obſervation will apply to rheumatiſm, compared to the dropſy, and to many other diſeaſes.

There are between eighty and ninety diſeaſes and caſualties enumerated in the London bills, which, in the ſubſequent comments, I have diſentangled into their ſeparate genera. This will operate as a check and correction to the public regiſters; and by this, their defects and errors will be apparent. But objections and difficulties occur in our reſearches for collateral information and illuſtration from hoſpital records. The diſeaſes of hoſpitals are by no means a general ſtandard of the diſeaſes of the metropolis, and much leſs of the whole nation. The reaſons alſo are glaring, why, in hoſpitals, diſeaſes ſhould be leſs fatal; and in this reſpect, cities ſhould have the advantage of the country. We cannot therefore apply hoſpital regiſters as a general criterion to a nation, neither as to the meaſurement of diſeaſes, nor of cures. Whenever authentic and ſyſtematic records of diſeaſes, recovery, and mortality, are kept in hoſpitals, domeſtick as well as military, and annually publiſhed, whatever may be alledged reſpecting the importance and demerits of ſuch inſtitutions, the community, at all events, will derive much uſeful information. One fourth of the annual mortality of Paris is in hoſpitals. But in contraſting the ſucceſs of medical practice in different hoſpitals of Europe, criticks have forgot to aſcertain the diſeaſes which are admitted or excluded, and the proportion of the former; conſequently their inferences are imperfect and erroneous.

CHAP.

CHAP IV.

FEVERS: amongſt the moſt univerſal and fatal maladies of our metropolis and iſland are *fevers*, with which I begin this morbid ſurvey. The principal and moſt general febrile epidemicks which infeſted England during two centuries, are enumerated in a ſhort abſtract, by Dr. Short; and conſiſt of plagues, agues, remittent fevers, ſummer and autumnal dyſenteries, ſpotted putrid fevers, ſlow fevers, ſmall-pox, meaſles, putrid and contagious peripneumonies, fatal ſpring pleuriſies, and peripneumonies, and epidemical catarrhs. Great national calamities, however, from this ſource, are rare: none ever inundate a whole kingdom (catarrh in ſome inſtances excepted): they ſometimes indeed ſpread from one province to another, but all the community are never attacked at once; nor are large populous kingdoms, or even cities, totally exempt from them. Fevers of various generic forms, may be local and circumſcribed to one city or diſtrict, whilſt others in the vicinity, continue at the ſame time healthy; the diſeaſe diſſipating its virulence within a ſmall boundary.

The abſolute mortality by fevers in the London bills, without including the ſmall-pox and meaſles, amounts to nearly one *ſeventh* of the whole funeral catalogue. In the London diſpenſaries, the Alderſgate and Weſtminſter, and in the Newcaſtle hoſpital, fevers were a fourth and ſixth to all other diſeaſes. De Haen computes,

putes, that out of two thouſand ſick, admitted into the hoſpitals in Vienna, ſeven hundred of them laboured under acute and febrile diſeaſes. Dr. Cleghorn eſtimates the ſummer fevers in Minorca, as conſtituting three-fourths of all the diſeaſes in that iſland. Dr. Lind calculates, that nineteen out of twenty deaths of all the Europeans who viſit the ſultry climates of Africa, America, and of the Eaſt and Weſt Indies, muſt be imputed to intermittent, remittent fevers, and fluxes; and probably he alſo ſhould have added, or to chronic diſeaſes and broken conſtitutions, the conſequence of thoſe fevers.

In the London bills of mortality, many different genera of fevers are crammed into one indiſcriminate heap, from which it is impoſſible to extricate the ſpecific nature or genus of febrile carnage. I was anxious to determine with ſome probability, the ratio of deſolation in London, by each of the different febrile genera; becauſe it would be an important guide to the prevention and cure. I knew that moſt of our hoſpital regiſters were in this particularly defective: on that account I was favoured by a medical friend with the peruſal of the books of the Alderſgate Diſpenſary. But although no gentlemen are better qualified to diſcriminate diſeaſes, I perceived, on inſpection, that too often the genus of fevers was not marked, only by the general outlines of the claſs. However, I converted this ſcrutiny to ſome other uſe, as will hereafter appear.

Intermitting fevers, or agues. It would ſeem, by the London regiſters, that very few die of agues, from which no age is exempted, but to

which

which adults are much more obnoxious than youth. Intermittent havock, if not immediately, yet in its chronic effects, is far more fatal than the London bills represent. Towns in general, it is true, are less harrassed with agues than country places. Pringle remarks, that during the campaigns of the British troops in the marshy countries of Holland and Flanders, where, in all such climates, and in damp soils and situations, agues and remittent fevers are epidemick, that the soldiers quartered in towns were less afflicted than those stationed in country cantonments: that in the former, the fires, sewers, drains and paved streets, prevented an exuberance of moisture: and that, if the men slept in the upper floors of the house, they were still more secure from damp and intermittent sickness.

Intermittent fevers are usually distinguished into different genera, or types; into quotidian, tertian, quartan, with their separate species and varieties. The invasion of intermittent paroxisms is during certain periods only, and generally consists of a successive series of shivering and cold, burning heat, profuse sweats, accelerated pulse, disordered stomach, head-ach, prostration of strength; and exhibits the fundamental outlines of all fevers. Intermittent paroxisms, and consequently the genera and species, vary in recurrence, in duration, and in the symptoms. Quotidians, tertians, and quartans, consist of paroxisms, at the respective intervals of 24, 48, and 72 hours. Each paroxism is terminated in less than 24 hours; the hot and sweating stages constituting the greatest portion of ſuch radical conflict: and of which the quotidian is the longeſt, the quartan the ſhorteſt.

Again, the type of intermittents is often obſcured under a cloud of irregular and adventitious ſymptoms; and from one predominant ſymptom, or from ſimilarity to various other diſeaſes, theſe three fundamental genera are ſplit by Noſologiſts into other ſpecies and varieties; the quotidiana, or intermittens, into ſimplex, cephalalgica, ophthalmica, nephralgica, ſtranguriosa, iſchiadica, ſputatoria, catarrhalis, anginoſa, epileptica, hyſterica, partialis: the tertiana into ſimplex, hemitritæa, duplex, triplex, pleuritica, aſthmatica, arthritica, emetica, hyſterica, apoplectica, urticata, and other ſpecies of double tertian enumerated under the remittent type: the quartana into cataleptica, epileptica, hyſterica, maniaca, comatoſa, nephralgica, ſplenetica, arthritica. Beſides, from various natural or accidental cauſes the type of intermittents may be changed: the quartan and tertian into quotidian; the latter into remittent, and theſe again into continued fever.

Notwithſtanding their febrile type, intermittents fall under the chronic claſs of diſeaſes. Vernal agues are ſaid not to be ſo refractory as the autumnal; nor the quotidian and tertian, as the quartan. But in young ſound conſtitutions, agues, if not inveterate, are frequently cured after a few paroxiſms. When death happens in them, it is generally during the cold ſtage, or vital collapſe. More frequently their fatality is by tranſition into ſome other chronic diſeaſes; ſuch as maladies of the ſtomach, digeſtive

geſtive organs, liver, and inteſtinal tube, bilious cachexy, jaundice, conſumption, dropſy.

Remitting fevers: fevers with remiſſions and exacerbations, or which have not, like the preceding, a temporary and total ceſſation, are the moſt univerſal febrile form in all parts of the globe. Throughout the equatorial oven, or middle regions of the earth, from cancer to capricorn, intermittents, but, above all, remittents and dyſenteries are the moſt univerſal type of fever. They are the locuſts which devour whole corps of mankind. During the periodical rainy ſeaſons of the tropical zones; particularly where they are choaked up with woods and moraſſes, and in uncultivated new ſettlements, theſe fevers often ravage with the deſolation of an Egyptian peſtilence; and are ſometimes ſo precipitate as to kill in one or two paroxiſms, if not ſooner repulſed; the doctor, lawyer, and prieſt quickly ſucceeding each other in their viſits. They deſtroy not only multitudes immediately, eſpecially of the new European ſettlers, ſoldiers and ſailors; but when improperly treated, or when convaleſcents from irregularity, fall back into relapſes, they often terminate in fatal chronic diſeaſes, ſimilar to thoſe recently enumerated under the intermittent train.

Not only within the tropicks, but likewiſe through the northern hemiſphere, to the verge nearly of the polar circles, we can deſcry this remittent febrile hoſt. In the ſultry ſummer and autumnal ſeaſons of Europe, in low marſhy countries, ſoils and ſituations ſuch as Italy and Hungary, where the ſummers are long and intenſe, and in that northern moraſs, Holland, theſe

theſe are the epidemical tyrants. Armies encamped are often at that ſeaſon grievouſly infeſted with them, and with dyſenteric fluxes. In Britain and Ireland alſo, they are frequent and fatal epidemicks; and are not confined to the ſummer ſeaſon only. Even in moſt dry countries and ſituations without the tropicks, after an unuſual cloſe ſultry ſummer, with long protracted heats, we often ſee, or read of, ſuch fevers and fluxes. The humours then, ſays Pringle, are corrupted, the ſolids relaxed; and in ſuch a diſpoſition of body, irregularities in diet, wet cloaths, and damp air, may give activity to ſuch latent indiſpoſition. In that ſmall Mediterranean iſland, as deſcribed by Cleghorn, where the ſoil is rocky, but the ſummer heats exceſſive, ſuch fevers have raged with atrocious ſeverity.

Fevers intermittent and remittent, and thoſe ſtrictly ſimple inflammatory, are greatly regulated, not only by the climate, latitude, ſoil, local elevation or depreſſion, but alſo in the ſame country by the different ſeaſons of the year. In ſummer and autumn, fevers tend in various degrees to affect the ſtomach and inteſtines with ſickneſs; they are then, more or leſs remittent, and participate leſs of the inflammatory. We may alſo add, that in all warm climates and ſeaſons there is a copious and ſuperabundant ſecretion of bile, and that none of the animal fluids ſo ſoon turn putrid. "In Holland,"[2] continues Pringle, "towards June, a healthy "month, the inflammatory fevers begin to re- "cede; and the remittent, bilious, and putrid "often ſucceed throughout the ſummer and

"autumn

" autumn, until the return of winter, when the " inflammatory again recommence; the ſeaſons " and diſeaſes inſenſibly interchanging and run- " ning into each other." But againſt this aphoriſm of Dr. Pringle's, we ſhall preſently have occaſion to expreſs our diſſent. They are more obnoxious to remittent fevers who are conſtantly exerciſed in labour and fatigue, and expoſed to the external air, than other ranks who are comfortably accommodated, cloathed, and fed. Pringle remarks, that the peaſants of Holland were always greater ſufferers by the ſummer, autumnal, and remittent fevers, than thoſe of the more opulent claſs; and alſo, that during ſummer and winter, in the field and in garriſon, the private ſoldiers were more ſickly and liable to fevers than the officers.

Remittent fevers ſeem to conſiſt of a repetition of protracted diurnal paroxiſms, or periodical aggravated exacerbations, nearly ſimilar to the intermittent or primitive type; but without the latter's complete intermiſſion. Authors have deſcribed them under a variety of apellations; but they may be all comprehended as ramifications of one great trunk, or integral genus: they appear in eſſence the ſame diſeaſe, and are cured by ſimilar remedies. In the medical nomenclature, they are denominated remittent, ſemitertian, hemitritea, tritophyea, double and triple tertian, putrid remittent, marſh, camp, ardent, bilious fevers, gall ſickneſs; tertian fever obſcured under a miſt of one or more of the following dangerous and prominent ſymptoms, hence named lethargick, vertiginous, ſoporoſe, apoplectick, paralytick, cata-

leptick,

leptick, epileptick, convulſive, phrenitick, hyſterick, ſyncopale, aſthmatick, arthritick, cardialgick, ſingultuous, rheumatick, pleuritick, dyſenterick, bilious, atrabilarian, cholerick, emetick, diaphoretick, pituitous, miliary, ſcorbutick.

Excluſive of the ſymptoms common to ſuch fevers, and partly delineated under the intermittent paroxiſm, remittent fevers are variouſly diverſified by a rotine and medley of nervous, putrid, and inflammatory ſymptoms; but with infinitely more of the two former. The climate, ſeaſon of the year, remiſſions, and the notorious epidemick or endemick of that region or place, all contribute to their unerring detection. Sometimes they attack very ſuddenly and violently with delirium and inflammatory ſimulation; but ſoon afterwards, and at the interval of a few days, remiſſions are evident. Sometimes, on the other hand, their approach is in appearance mild, but not leſs alarming. According to Lind, the tropical remittents are the moſt virulent, yet are not contagious, unleſs accompanied with dyſentery, or the ſick crowded together; which, if an irrefragable fact, diſtinguiſhes this fever from the nervous and putrid: and beſides, in the febrile epidemicks and endemicks, from marſhy effluvia, the remiſſions are more perceptible and ſynchronous than in theſe from animal contagion. From the air, ſeaſon, and medical treatment, the remittent may be converted into the continued or intermittent type: in the latter there is more ſecurity. In warm climates putreſcency and death

may

may enſue in a few paroxiſms; in others, in all the intervals during three weeks.

The prediſpoſing and occaſional cauſes of intermittent and remittent fevers are, cloudy winter and autumn; northern moraſſes: noxious miaſma or emanations from moraſſes; and from countries and ſoils low, damp, rank, woody, uncultivated, more eſpecially in warm climates, weather, and ſeaſons; moiſt and hot atmoſphere; foggy atmoſphere; unuſual irregularity of the ſeaſons and atmoſphere; unuſual continuance of cold rainy weather; damp night air, eſpecially in warm unhealthy climates; exceſſive heats; burning zones and regions; ſudden viciſſitudes from heat to cold of the ſeaſons and weather; unuſually exceſſive and long continued heats; damp weather, particularly when, at the ſame time, it is unuſually warm for the ſeaſon and climate; dampy ground floors and habitations; damp ſheets and beds; ſleeping in the open air and on damp ground, eſpecially with the head uncovered; ſudden ſtoppage of perſpiration; depraved, redundant bile; ſeptic miaſma, introduced from without, or generated within the body; efforts of nature to diſencumber its functions and organs of ſome clogs and impurities. Perhaps rather contributing as exciting cauſes are paſſions of mind, fatigue, hardſhips, long watching, hunger, thirſt, intoxication, venery to exceſs, interruption of the excretions.

Nervous and Putrid Fevers have been deſcribed under various names: under ſlow nervous fevers, nervous and putrid fevers, the ſlow treacherous malignant, putrid remittent, camp, jail, hoſpital, infectious, putrid, malignant, continued,

tinued, ſpotted, purple, petechial, yellow fevers, &c. This febrile hoſt are alſo widely diſperſed over the earth; and probably are not ſo much governed or influenced as the preceding remittents by the climate, ſeaſon, and ſenſible qualities of the atmoſphere; but may originate in all countries, climates, ſeaſons, and ſituations; and when extremely virulent, may, like the plague or ſmall-pox, be communicated by imperceptible emanation or contagion from one infected perſon to another, by perſonal intercourſe, by the medium of polluted goods, furniture, apparel, cloaths, and houſes; in all which the noxious miaſma may be concentrated and lodged. Sometimes they harraſs a nation or city in detachment only; and ſometimes in formidable phalanx. Such fevers are frequently engendered in jails, crowded with filth and animal ſteams, and excluded from free ventilation; alſo in military hoſpitals, crammed with ſick, and with dyſenteries, putrid ſores, and mortifications; alſo in ſhips and large fleets, when haſtened out in the hurry and ſpur of approaching hoſtilities; alſo in wet and ſtormy weather at ſea, when the hatches are cloſed.

In cities, contagious fevers may be traced to priſons, perhaps ſometimes to hoſpitals; certainly often to narrow courts and alleys, and ſmall crowded apartments; to the houſes of the indigent; to filth, rags, and ſqualid poverty, co-operating with foul unventilated air: and in the open perflated ſtreets, are much leſs frequent. Cities, therefore, ſhould be more infeſted with them than the country; and the poor more than the affluent. Children, with adults are

are ſubject to them, but prodigiouſly more of the latter. Some, not without argument, alledge, that ſlow nervous and putrid fevers are in general derived from the ſame origin; and that they differ from each other in degree only. Petechial ſpots are by no means conſtant ſymptoms of the putrid type; but when they occur, they point out the diſeaſe more unerringly, and its greater malignity. In many inſtances, their differences may be rationally imputed to climate, ſeaſon, conſtitution, miaſma, and medical treatment.

I meet with inextricable embarraſſment, in endeavouring to draw the exact limits, not only between nervous and putrid fevers, but alſo between them and what ſome authors have termed the univerſal remittent of this iſland; and which is not limitted to any ſeaſon of the year. I take this opportunity, therefore, to avow, that in what proportion theſe very general fevers with remiſſions originate from marſhy effluvia, from climate, and conſtitutional indiſpoſition, from animal contagion, or from other occult cauſes, I am unable to decide: their preciſe relation as to lineage and conſanguinity, is beyond my penetration.

Slow nervous fever frequently ſteals on with treacherous mildneſs; the ſick are rendered unfit for buſineſs, but yet not confined to bed, and except to ſagacious judges, the fever is not apparently alarming; and too often the ſick and their friends are lulled into fatal ſecurity. The prominent features are fever, inappetency, diſordered ſtomach; the functions of the brain, the nervous and muſcular energy, in a word, the corporeal

corporeal and mental functions considerably weakened and interrupted. The remissions are generally more distinct in the beginning, and by degrees become more obscure. Putrid fever sometimes also creeps on with deceitful approach under the nervous cloak; and sometimes, with furious onset, counterfeits the inflammatory. As to the term malignant, it may be applied to most fevers, when accompanied with dangerous symptoms. In the duration, crisis, and termination of nervous and putrid fevers, there is considerable diversity. Some may be suddenly stifled before they burst into a flame: some of inveterate malignity may prove fatal in a few days; others may terminate in all the intervals within three weeks, and later. Some terminate auspiciously, without any sensible crisis or evacuation: in others, there is more or less sensible defecation by some of the large excretories. The dangerous symptoms in each of these fevers are hereafter pointed out under the general synopsis of febrile prognosticks.

The predisposing and occasional causes of nervous and putrid fevers are, many, or perhaps all of the preceding causes of intermittents or remittents: noxious miasma or contagion, engendered from human effluvia in cities, jails, hospitals, ships, small crowded houses and apartments, especially in unventilated alleys, lanes, and courts: accumulation of corporeal filth and perspiration, from want of cloathing, change of raiment, slothfulness: contagion concentrated in porous materials, furniture, raiment, houses, and ships: cadaverous exhalations, effluvia from putrid carcasses of animals, and from animal

and

and vegetable heaps in a ſtate of putrid fermentaion, and from putrid ſores and mortifications; gangrenous inoculation through wounds of the ſkin; damp, rainy ſeaſons; bad harveſt and putrid grain; putrid diet, animal or farinaceous; improper medical treatment of remittent fevers; corrupted bile, or other ſecreted and excreted fluids, noxious in quantity or quality; profuſe evacuations; immoderate venery; deſponding paſſions of mind; intemperance in food or drink; ſtoppage of perſpiration.

Miliary fever, febris purpurata, rubra and alba, is never epidemick, and is denied to be a primary diſeaſe; but is ſpurious, ſymptomatick, acceſſary, or fortuitous: it is very rare, and may be complicated with the nervous and putrid fever, and with ſmall-pox and meaſles. The miliaris alba is more frequent amongſt the female ſex, eſpecially during the puerperal ſtate, and in other females debilitated by fluor albus, and hemorrhages, of weak conſtitutions, delicate, prolifick; and ſometimes exhibits previous ſymptoms of angina, pleuriſy, catarrh, rheumatiſm, eryſipelas. Its peculiar diagnoſticks are extreme debility and ſinking of all the mental and corporeal functions, and of muſcular energy; a cutaneous puſtular, prurient effloreſcence, emitting a peculiar ſour ſmell, and frequently a retroceſſion and new eruption; and without morbillous ſternutation.

The prediſpoſing and occaſional cauſes of miliary fever are, eſtuation, hot regimen and rooms, during fever and parturition; exceſſive evacuations, weak conſtitution, debility, depreſſing paſſions, moiſt air, wet ſummer.

Inflammatory Fevers, ſynochus continua non putris of Boerhaave. To this we may add the febris diaria. A different genus of fever, both in its nature and cure, from the remittent, nervous, and putrid, is the ſimple inflammatory. The frequency and the fatality of this fever, is infinitely inferior to the preceding groups; and in compariſon, is as the ſpoliation of an Algerine pirate to the devaſtation of a Tamerlane. Pringle obſerves, that in military camps, pleuriſies, and peripnuemonies are the moſt frequent form of fever with inflammation; and next to theſe acute rheumatiſms. The predominancy and reign of inflammatory fever, is in cold climates and rigorous ſeaſons, in the winter and ſpring of northern latitudes, and where cold and moiſture are combined. It commonly attacks the robuſt, ſtrong, athletick, and thoſe in the vigour of life: it is not contagious; and neither its remiſſion nor exacerbation are conſpicuous. Its aſſault is ſudden and violent, with a ſtrong, full pulſe, accelerated reſpiration, intenſe heat of the ſkin, thirſt, and head-ach. But in general the mental functions are not ſo greatly diſordered, nor the muſcular debility ſo great as in the nervous and putrid fevers. Its termination is uſually in the interval between four and eleven days.

The prediſpoſing and occaſional cauſes of inflammatory, and of tranſitory or diary fevers are, cold climates and winter; cold winds; change of the ſeaſons; heat of the atmoſphere; inſolation; exceſſive labour; exceſſive fatigue; violent paſſions of mind; long watching; cold drink when the body is heated; intoxication with

with ſpirituous liquors; crude chyle; heating ſtimulating diet; diſordered foul ſtomach; plethora; exceſs of coagulable lymph and its tenacity; menſtrual, lacteal, hemorrhoidal, arthritick, excruciating pains; warm baths.

With reſpect to all the preceding confederate genera of fevers, we ſhall make the following general obſervations. In the preceding century, during the laſt thirty years, febrile mortality, by the London bills, is rated at 87,645: and the mortality of the preſent century is ſeen in the Chart of London diſeaſes. Formerly, in this metropolis and iſland, and probably throughout Europe, fevers ſeem to have been much more prevalent and fatal than at preſent: their cauſes, eſſential nature, and cure, is now much better underſtood by phyſicians; and we are provided with far more powerful auxiliary remedies, and are more expert in their application. In this particular inſtance, modern medicine, eſpecially of the century in which we live, is ſignalized, and may, without arrogance, claim triumphal honours. The ſuppoſed innumerable varieties of fevers, and from which perplexity Sydenham could not altogether extricate himſelf, is now diſproved by repeated experience, and by the infallible efficacy of general remedies. It is, however, as yet impoſſible to fix any definite medium or average of mortality in the above genera of fevers, whether remittent, nervous, putrid, or inflammatory. We have, within theſe few years, authentick records, wherein, under judicious and ſkilful treatment, of 200 ſick in both remittent, nervous, and putrid fevers, only one or two *per cent.* died.

Nor was this ſucceſs confined to European climates only; but extended through the tropical regions: whereas, under different and erroneous management, one half, and often the greateſt part of the ſick periſhed. The proof of theſe aſſertions may be ſeen in thoſe learned authors, Lind, Millar, Robinſon, Clarke, Lettſom, Sims, and others.

Not only in London, but throughout Britain, and throughout the globe, perhaps nine tenths of the fevers are of the remittent, nervous, and putrid type, and not of the ſimple inflammatory. But I exclude from this calculation the following exanthematous order, and the topical inflammations. The falſe lights hung out ſucceſſively by multitudes of authors, and tranſmitted, in ſome degree, through the Boerhaavean ſchool, to ſteer with the antiphlogiſtick compaſs and lancet in each hand, in the generality of fevers, have been the cauſe of numerous ſhipwrecks. Even that excellent modern author, Pringle, as Dr. Millar demonſtrates, muſt, in this inſtance, be followed with extreme caution.

Throughout the intire morbid hoſt of human foes, there is probably no ſuch flagrant variation in the therapeutick barometer, or ſcale of mortality, as in that of the fevers hitherto deſcribed. Different curatory proceſſes and remedies ſoon change the natural genus, ſymptoms, criſis, prognoſticks, and event. No dangerous diſeaſes almoſt whatſoever, are more ſucceſsfully oppugnable under diſcreet medical regimen; and when entruſted to nature, from the days of Hippocrates to the preſent time, they have ever been extremely fatal. Sorry I

am

am to add, that, perhaps in many inſtances, the errors and fatality of nature, have been leſs deſtructive than thoſe of artificial and therapeutick miſmanagement. Since the diſcovery of antimonials and Peruvian bark, the more liberal uſe of wine, and freſh air, and more ſparing exerciſe of the lancet, few now, under ſkilful medical pilots, die, compared to the multitudes of ſick: but ſtill in the aggregate liſt of funerals, amounting to 780,000 annually in Europe, it may be doubted whether any other of the morbid foes commit ſuch ravages amongſt mankind.

The ruin of armies and navies during actual hoſtilities, from the earlieſt ages to the preſent time, and throughout every quarter of the globe, is to be aſcribed principally to the preceding fevers, together with dyſentery and ſcurvy. We muſt ſearch the regiſters of military hoſpitals, and not of the field of battle, for the deſtruction and rot of warriors. This I ſhall prove to demonſtration hereafter, when treating on the comparative deſtruction of the human ſpecies in conſequence of war. But what is ſtill more ſhocking to humanity, the greateſt part of this morbid carnage is to be imputed to the ignorance or miſconduct of the different rulers of mankind, and to their military and medical generals.

Small-Pox, natural and inoculated. We have no veſtiges, neither in hiſtory nor tradition, of this loathſome diſeaſe, nor of the meaſles, before the irruption of Mahomet and his followers from the Arabian deſerts, about 1,300 years ago; and from whom this extraneous contagion was firſt tranſplanted into Europe. It is little

 more

more than 200 years ſince the exportation of this exotic poiſon to the American continent, where it had never before been ſeen nor heard of. The havock by this ſcourge of the human race, amounts, in London, to nearly a decimation of the inhabitants; and to 494,000 annually, throughout Europe. It is equally or oftener much more fatal throughout the torrid and frigid zones; and in the adult age is more violent than in childhood. It attacks the ſame perſon but once in life: had this not been the caſe, the human race muſt long ſince have been extinct. On a promiſcuous average, one of every ſeven infected die of the natural diſeaſe; but under inoculation only 1 of 500. Beſides, to the former deadly catalogue may be ſuperadded a frightful train of mangled conſtitutions, and countenances, of conſumptions, abſceſſes, ulcers, opthalmies, blindneſs.

In every large metropolis, ſmall-pox is an annual epidemick. In country towns and open diſtricts, its invaſions are more diſtant; at uncertain intervals of ſome years, when numbers contiguous are attacked at the ſame time. In our climate, it is alledged to be moſt prevalent in ſpring and autumn. Very few of the human ſpecies eſcape the ſmall pox, eſpecially in populous cities and towns, wherein there is always laſting variolous fuel, or lurking embers: it might eaſily be demonſtrated, that in London, and probably in all other large cities, variolous ravages are principally amongſt children under five years of age. Without entering into any elaborate argumentation, or proofs of this aſſertion, the reader may, in ſome degree, be convinced,

vinced, by only turning his eye to our firſt Chart, and to a ſmall contiguous table of London mortality during ten years; wherein he will obſerve the trifling annual mortality in the interval between 5 and 20 years: before which laſt period, a mere handful of the native progeny of the metropolis can be ſuppoſed to have eſcaped an infection with which they are conſtantly enveloped. It is obvious that the total annual mortality by all diſeaſes, incluſively, in London during this adoleſcent period of life of 15 years, is not equal to variolous carnage ſingly. As to inoculation, or artificial engrafting of the contagion, it is throughout the greateſt part of Europe a modern practice of the preſent century, and is yet in its cradle. Even in the London ſmall-pox hoſpital, ſince its firſt inſtitution, forty years ago, there have not been inoculated altogether 25,000.

The cruel carnage perpetrated by ſmall-pox throughout the earth; the rooted prejudices, and the inſinuations urged to ſhackle the univerſal benefits of inoculation, and which pervade not only the ignorant maſs of the community, but alſo the generality of the medical profeſſion throughout Europe, would abundantly excuſe and urge me to be more diffuſe on this intereſting and litigated topick. But having, ſome years ago, publiſhed a ſmall Eſſay on the advantages and diſadvantages of early Inoculation, and having now nearly finiſhed a general treatiſe on the natural and inoculated ſmall-pox, I ſhall poſtpone the reſult of much reading and reflection to that republication. An acquieſcence in neutrality or indifference, where it can be proved to mathematical demonſtration that myriads of lives might be preſerved, which are now ſacrificed, would, at leaſt in a moral ſenſe, conſtitute an acceſſary in criminality.

Small-pox, or variolæ, have been properly diſcriminated into ſeveral ſpecies: the diſtinct and confluent, or benign and malign; the cryſtalline, lymphatick, warty, petechial, and hemorrhagick; the inoculated; the ſpurious. Formerly indeed, ſmall-pox, naturally mild, were often rendered malignant by confined air, heated chambers, and regimen. The principal differences between ſmall-pox conſiſt in the period of eruption, the number and form of the puſtules, the quantity and ſtate of the fluid contained in them, and the contumacious perſeverance of the fever. The progreſs of variolous fever has been divided into four ſtages, that preceding the eruption; the eruption; the ſuppuration; and the exſiccation of the puſtules. The three firſt ſtages are uſually compleated within ten or eleven days from the firſt attack, when, at leaſt in the mild form of the diſeaſe, the maturated puſtules begin to dry and ſhrivel.

The following are all unfavourable ſymptoms in ſmall-pox: ſudden and premature eruption of puſtules; epileptick fits; puſtules numerous or confluent, eſpecially on the face; puſtules hard or warty; the puſtules not ſufficiently diſtended and filled, watery, in flat coaleſcent veſicles, or not filled with yellow, maturated, and concocted pus; the top of the puſtules depreſſed; pale interſtices at their baſe, ſudden retroceſſion or ſubſidence of the puſtules, during the ſtage of maturation; cutaneous pete-

chiæ

chiæ interſperſed; bloody puſtules; the fever continuing throughout pertinaceous, and without remiſſion, and with putreſcency its danger is aggravated; ſevere inflammation of the fauces; difficult deglutition; acute pain at the ſtomach; putrid urine; emphyſematous abdomen; the fever continuing to rage during the ſuppurating ſtage, the ſalivation then ceaſing, and not ſucceeded by ſwelling of the hands. The ſecondary fever ariſing commonly, or more properly increaſing about the period of receſſion and exſiccation of the puſtules, or ebb of maturation, is the moſt dangerous ſtage in ſmall-pox. The criſis and defecation of the floating pus is then by diarrhœa, urine, or ſalivation. When the putreſcency is very virulent, the diſeaſe ſometimes proves fatal in a few days; but in moſt caſes on the eleventh, and ſometimes not until the fourteenth or ſeventeenth.

Inoculated Small-Pox. In ninety-nine caſes out of an hundred, inoculation produces a diſtinct ſmall-pox, void of danger. The puſtules in general are not numerous; and the patients are ſeldom confined to bed, or indiſpoſed. After inoculation from maturated puſtules of real ſmall-pox, and the uſual ſymptoms of impregnation, mankind are ever after invulnerable by this contagion.

The ſuppoſition of a perſon undergoing the diſeaſe a ſecond time, either after the natural or inoculated ſmall-pox, originated from a ſpurious ſource, and what are called chicken, baſtard, petite verole volante, ſtein, and ſwain pox; which are ſometimes epidemick, but inoffenſive, and of a few days duration.

Meaſles.

Measles. Morbilli, rubeola. From 100 to 100 20th part of the community seem to be destroyed by measles. Morbillous mortality is to that of small-pox in the ratio of 1 to 10, or 12; and consequently may be estimated at 1 of 77 whom it attacks. Sydenham, long ago observed, that measles, if judiciously treated, are attended with very little danger: but he should at least have qualified the expression, by adding immediate and considerable danger; for both immediately, and in their future consequences, they are by no means so innocuous. Few escape this exotick contagion, especially in childhood and in cities. It attacks the same person but once in life; and, with us, is said to be most epidemick in winter.

This cutaneous efflorescence resembles the bites of ants, and is generally confluent and entangled: it never rises into prominent pustules, nor suppurates; and within nine days from the first attack of the fever is obliterated. Unfavourable symptoms are, too sudden or too tardy eruption; pale or yellow eruption; great debility; pertinacious fever and cough; and above all, pulmonick inflammation. The last in the train of morbillous evils and consequences are, consumption, anasarca, ophthalmy.

Scarlet Fever. Febris scarlatina, ignis sacer, scarlatina anginosa. Its mortality in the London bills is obscured amongst the general febrile heap. This contagious epidemick is most frequent in the infant and adolescent age; it attacks families and schools about one time; and the same person but once in life; and is said to be most frequent in wihter. It is generally accompanied

companied with an anginous or ulcerous ſore throat, but ſeldom putrid. That genus or ſpecies of ſcarlet fever which uſually accompanies the angina gangrenoſa, and which is extremely dangerous, is hereafter deſcribed. It is uſhered in by the uſual febrile precurſors, ſucceeded between two and four days by a cutaneous ſuperficial eruption, general or partial, over the face, and over various parts of the body and extremities; by diſordered ſtomach, and difficulty in deglutition. The criſis and termination of theſe complaints are uſually within nine days; by one or more of the larger excretories; and exſcreation of ſloughs. The dangerous and fatal ſymptoms are nearly ſimilar to thoſe of nervous and putrid fevers, and of gangrenous angina. Sometimes during the convaleſcent ſtate, from expoſure to cold air, or neglect of proper preventative remedies, dropſy has ſuddenly enſued.

Plague. Peſtis. This febrile demon cannot now be called one of the mortal epidemicks of Europe, except in the South-eaſt extremity, inhabited by the Turks. The two greateſt peſtilences on record, happened in the ſixth and fourteenth centuries of our era; by which millions in three quarters of the globe were overwhelmed in one indiſcriminate maſſacre. In London, before the general conflagration in 1666, of one half nearly of the old city, the plague was very frequent: but ſince that event, or at the moſt two or three years after, it has been exterminated and baniſhed from us. That fortunate diſaſter which conſumed a magazine of putrefaction; together with widened ſtreets, ventilation, cleanlineſs,

cleanlineſs, a more plentiful ſupply of water and many other cauſes, have all contributed to the extinction of this exotick incendiary. For it is well known, that peſtilential miaſma has been preſerved dormant many years in porous materials. From 1592 to 1665, the plague appears to have had annually more or leſs ſhare in the mortality of the Britiſh metropolis; and adding together the different periods of its duration, amounts to twenty-five years. In 1665, which is the moſt furious peſtilence in the London annals, the deaths amounted to 100,000; but in the eight preceding years, to only 113. Regiſters, in other parts of Europe, prove, that this diſeaſe has committed direful carnage ſince our emancipation. At Marſeilles they can enumerate twenty general plagues, which have ſucceſſively laid waſte that populous city. Many other European cities and towns, during the laſt and preſent century, and eſpecially thoſe bordering on the Mediterranean, have, in a very ſhort ſpace of time, ſeverely ſmarted by peſtilence, and have been nearly depopulated.

At preſent, in all the Mediterranean ports they are, from fatal experience, ſcrupulouſly vigilant to guard, by a circumvallation of alarm poſts, againſt the peſtilential infection, and the clandeſtine entry of infected goods or merchandize. It rarely now gains admittance, by ſtealth, into any of the European ports; (Conſtantinople excepted) or even if imported to our ſhores, the wiſe precautions and regulations, enacted by quarantines, ſoon check its irruption and progreſs. This is a moſt intereſting epoch and improvement in the police of modern ſtates;

for

for the original inftitution and rough draft of which, about 300 years ago, we are indebted to the Venetians. The political ordinances, however, enacted for the exclufion and fuppreffion of peftilential contagion, were, until the prefent century, extremely erroneous and impolitick. Formerly, the plague in London, and in moft other European cities, where it was permitted to fojourn, was rendered infinitely more terrifick and deftructive by injudicious legiflative regulations; efpecially by the barbarous and abfurd policy of immuring the fick and found together, with a forlorn motto on their doors, until all were dead or recovered. This was an effectual difcouragement againft an early alarm, which, as in cafes of fire, is of the utmoft importance. It is evident, by the London bills, that a mere handful, at any time, died in the publick peft-houfe; confequently, every corner of the city was polluted with infection.

True plague is now chiefly circumfcribed to Conftantinople, and to Grand Cairo in Egypt, the two original, or at leaft one of the hot-beds and volcanos of peftilence; to feveral of the maritime towns of Afia and Africa, fituated on the Archipelago and Mediterranean; as Smyrna, Aleppo, Tripoli, Tunis, Algiers, &c. In many of thefe cities the peftilential miafma is hatched and accumulated into venomous malignity: it is in fome nearly an annual, or triennial epidemick. At this day, the plague almoft folely wreaks its venom on the Mahometan nations, whofe prejudices and ignorance, rivetted by religious and predeftinarian abfurdities, give licence and activity to its imperious domination.

Fortunately

Fortunately for mankind, the peſtilential contagion ſpreads to a very ſmall diſtance through the air, without ſome contact or adheſion to infected goods, porous materials; or by perſonal communication and intercourſe of the ſound with the diſeaſed. The atmoſphere is not tainted to any conſiderable diſtance. A neighbour barricading himſelf within his houſe, at a few yards diſtance from infection, may eſcape unhurt. If peſtilential contagion could be ſo ſuddenly and widely ſcattered over a kingdom as epidemical influenza, the earth, in a few months, would be converted into an enormous churchyard. It is not like ſome other exotick poiſons of the exanthematous order, after enduring which once, mankind are rendered invulnerable: the plague, as well as putrid fever, may attack the ſame perſon repeatedly.

The progreſſive peſtilential ſymptoms are great abaſement of the ſtrength and ſpirits, with nauſea, vomiting and head-ach: but its invariable characteriſtick features are, external buboes, carbuncles, and petechiæ. What proportion die or recover, I cannot aſcertain; and indeed the prophylactick or preventative, is infinitely the moſt important indication. According to the virulence of the contagion, and other cooperating cauſes, the diſeaſe may be fatal in a few hours, a few days, or in one, two, or three weeks. The poiſon arreſted in the external lymphatick glands and ſuppurating, is a favourable, gangrene and hemorrhages, a fatal preſage. Domeſtick animals, ſuch as quadrupeds and fowls, are alſo liable to the infection, and to be changed into carrion.

The

The predifpofing and occafional caufes of the plague are venomous effluvia, in certain hot climates, from putrid animal exhalations and filth; fuch as the ftagnant canals and refervoirs of putridity in Grand Cairo; putrid emanations from fwarms of dead locufts; from infection attached to moveable materials. The predifpofing caufes are, long watching, hunger, or poor diet, intemperance, excefs of venery, fatigue, terror, fear, debility, low fpirits, &c.

Sweating Sicknefs, ephemera fudatoria et elodes, cannot now be confidered as an epidemick caufe of mortality. Somewhat more than 300 years ago, this fingular contagious and vagrant difeafe, accompanied with profufe fweats, extreme debility, and ficknefs, burft out, for the firft time, in the army of Henry VII. in his return to England from an expedition againft France; and in four hours ficknefs, numbers were exterminated: but by keeping warm in bed, under profufe fweats, the dangerous whirlpool generally was efcaped. The fame infection was imported into England at feveral fubfequent intervals; but happily, its greateft devaftation was always of fhort duration; and this morbid meteor has long fince difappeared from our ifland, and from Europe. Sometimes it was fatal in one day; but, if the fick furvived to the feventh, they generally recovered.

With refpect to the great *fources* of fevers, noxious miafma from moraffes, contagion from human effluvia, and animal bodies, and that from fpecifick unknown origin, I fhall make a few obfervations. Of what elementary nature miafma and contagion confift; the analyfis of their

their minute atoms, whether animalcules, or to us inviſible emanations, I pretend not to decide. Still leſs do I pretend to pry into thoſe latent prediſpoſitions in the human organization, which render ſome more than others ſuſceptible to various febrile impreſſions. Of ſmall-pox, meaſles, ſcarlet fever, and ſweating ſickneſs, we are totally ignorant of their origin and eſſence: the two firſt are exotick leavens. We, however, know to a certainty, and it is of infinitely more importance to the publick ſafety, that neither marſhy miaſma, nor thoſe from human effluvia, ſpread to any conſiderable diſtance through the air. Even by the plague the atmoſphere is tainted to a very inconſiderable diſtance; and mankind find an aſylum and ſanctuary within a few yards. Nor do marſhy miaſma, emitted from the earth, mount or diffuſe themſelves to any conſiderable diſtance in the air: the inhabitants at the ſummit of a hill have continued healthy, whilſt thoſe ſituated in a ſwamp at the bottom, have been infeſted with intermittents, and remittents. To what diſtance the contagion of ſmall-pox, meaſles, and ſcarlet fever extend through the air, I am ignorant: like the plague, the two former have been tranſplanted to diſtant regions, in animal bodies, or in polluted porous materials. Another important diſcovery of modern times is, that by fire and ſmoke, the heat of a baker's oven, the moſt virulent contagion may be annihilated, when concentrated in apparel, ſpungy materials, ſhips, houſes, &c. in all which contagion may lay a length of time concealed.

Of

Of Febrile Prognosticks. The event of all the preceding fevers (intermittent excepted) is terminated with precipitancy in a few days, or, at the utmost, a few weeks, in recovery, in death, or in some other disease. The predictions in fevers, and indeed in all other diseases, should be deduced from the comparative mortality at different ages; the comparative mortality by different fevers; the specifick symptoms peculiar to each genus, whether ominous or propitious; and the general symptoms applicable to an intire group or class.

We have already treated, in regular progression, of the three former fundamental elements of prognosticks; reserving however, for this place, the ominous presages of remittent, nervous, and putrid fevers. At the same time the general prognosticks of danger in fevers, comprizing a concatenation of few or many of the following symptoms, may, in some degree, be transposed to the intire febrile class; even to the order of topical inflammations not yet surveyed.

It is foreign to my plan, to squander time or words, in eulogy or censure of those elaborate treatises on the pulse and urine, and their presumed extensive application to the diagnostick and prognostick of diseases. Of strength and weakness, hardness and softness, fulness and inanition, slowness, celerity, velocity, saliency, intermission, irregularity, and a few other distinctions of the circulation and arterial pulsation, we are competent judges; and of the measurement of velocity to a still greater nicety with the stop-watch. But, with all due reverence to Galen and his copyiſts, down to De Bordeu, in diſcriminating by touch the multitude and variety of complicated tones, combinations, diviſions, ſub-diviſions, chromaticks and chords in the arterial vibrations, we confeſs the bluntneſs and incapacity of our organs. Beſides, in the velocity of the pulſe prodigious variations enſue from age, ſex, conſtitution, temperament, climate, ſeaſon, food, drink, paſſions of mind, exerciſe, reſt, ſleep, waking, health, different diſeaſes, and different periods of the day.

We have ſtill fewer ſcruples to diſclaim that affected ſagacity and alchymiſtical intuition, of forming auguries, ſingly, from the urine; from its innumerable ſhades, intermixtures, pellicles, precipitation, and ſediment. This is, even in our time, one of the decoys in vaticination to inveigle the ignorant and credulous; the ſtale manœuvres and chiromancy of vagabond empiriciſm and impoſture. Nor ſhall we delay to comment upon the Hippocratic critical days in fevers; nor on the effects of the moon; both of which are more conſpicuous in topical climates.

We ſhall enumerate, in detail, the principal prognoſticks and ſymptoms of danger in fevers. The pulſe weak, quick, fluttering, ſalient, irregular, intermittent, its ſyſtole duplicated, its velocity 130 or 140; tendency to faint or fainting in an erect poſture; cold extremities; the reſpiration ſlow, laborious, quick, cold; all the ſubſidiary muſcles of reſpiration labouring to diſtend the thorax; deep interrupted ſighs, hiccup; particular noiſe in reſpiration, as if mucus plugged up the throat and lungs. The ſtomach

mach very weak, with extreme naufea, ficknefs, vomiting, defire of acids; thirft, deglutition difficult, ftruggling, and with noife; the tongue, teeth, and lips foul, and furred with a brown or black glutinous incruftation; more efpecially if after abfterfion it is quickly renewed: the urine pale, red, black, fetid; intenfe burning heat in the fkin, or in the abdomen; the belly tumid and puffed; involuntary excretion of feces and urine; fetid cadaverous feces, breath, and perfpiration; clammy fweats, efpecially on the breaft; the blood, if drawn, not coagulating; cutaneous petechiæ, like fmall bruifes in different parts; fubcutaneous effufions; hemorrhages; unremitting head-ach, vertigo, weaknefs, confufion, irregularity in the intellectual functions, finking of the fpirits, and defpondency; the manners different from natural; in the fpeech or actions fomething unufual; loquacity; no fleep, or not refrefhing; coma; delirium furious, or low and muttering; in the countenance and eyes perturbation, agitation, amazement, defpondency, defpair, anxiety, ftupefaction; attempts to rife out of bed; throwing off the bed-cloaths, inceffant toffing about the bed, reftleffnefs; forgetfulnefs, lofs of memory, fo as not to know the neareft friend; refufing or exfpuating food, drink, or medicines; moats floating before the eyes, and objects feen as through a cloud; total inattention to every object; twitching and fpafms of the tendons at the wrift; catching and picking with the hands and fingers at the bed-cloaths, as if feeling for fome object; ftarting of the mufcles, convulfions; trembling of the hands and tongue when thruſt out; ſupine poſture; great proſtration of ſtrength; inability to ſupport themſelves erect or ſitting; ſliding down to the foot of the bed; livid noſe; collapſed cheeks and temples; ſunk, glazy, and blood-ſhot eyes; inanimate, ghaſtly countenance.

The favourable termination of general fevers is chiefly diſcovered by ceſſation of delirium, abatement of the frequency of the pulſe; mild ſweats equally diffuſed; the urine depoſiting a ſediment freely and copiouſly; coolneſs of the ſkin; cleanneſs of the tongue; return of natural ſleep and appetite; and food recruiting the loſt ſtrength. The ſtorm is then ſubſided, and the ſhip arrived at anchor.

CHAP. V.

THE phlogiſtick group of febrile diſeaſes are now to be reviewed. The majority of theſe in their immediate cauſes and mode of cure, intimately anaſtomoſe; and the principal differences in the ſymptoms are to be aſcribed to the different organs and parts enraged by inflammation. Theſe are not like the generality of the preceding fevers, in which moſt of the corporeal functions participate: here, in many caſes, one ſingle portion of the human organization is originally transfixed with pain and commotion;

commotion; and doomed to bear the brunt of the hydraulick torrent and inundation. I avoid throughout the technical ſubtilties and diſtinction of parenchymatous and membranaceous inflammation. After mature conſideration, we imagined it would occaſion leſs confuſion and burthen to the memory, to detach a few diſeaſes from this group. Inflammations of the ears, eyes, inteſtines, kidneys, and bladder, are incorporated amongſt the other diſeaſes by which thoſe various organs are liable to be inveſted.

Inflammation of the Brain. Phrenitis vera. As a primary diſeaſe, it is very rare in this kingdom. It is much more frequent in tropical and hot climates: and is the febrile calenture of thoſe ſcorching regions. With us it is moſtly ſymptomatick in different fevers: and may either affect the brain and medullary ſubſtance, or its inveſting membranes. Morbid diſſections have proved, that when inflammation was believed to be preſent, none could be diſcovered; and in other caſes, that the brain was inflamed, without expreſſing the uſual ſymptoms: which are, excruciating head-ach, reſtleſſneſs, fever, delirium, wildneſs and ferocity of the eyes and countenance, intolerance of light and noiſe. It is extremely dangerous and precipitate, terminating in a few days in recovery, death, or ſome other diſeaſe; and is rarely protracted beyond a week: and on any irregularity or intemperance, convaleſcents are prone to relapſe.

The prediſpoſing and occaſional cauſes of phrenitis are, warm climate; inſolation, eſpecially with the head uncovered; ſudden ſuppreſſion of the puerperal lochia; intoxication;

violent paſſions of mind, ambition, anger, grief; profound contemplation, unremitting ſtudy; long deprivation of ſleep; external injuries; eryſipelas, or ſcald head prematurely repelled; violent exerciſe; ſymptomatick.

Angina: cynanche, quinſey; and diſtinguiſhed into the inflammatory; and into the putrid, gangrenous, or malignant. The mortality by quinſey and ſore throat, appears in the London bills inconſiderable; and without diſcrimination of the inflammatory and putrid. Inflammatory angina is a general and frequent affliction in both ſexes, and eſpecially in ours and ſome northern regions. Adults more than infants; and ſome individuals more than others, are obnoxious to it: its reign is in ſpring and autumn, on the change and viciſſitudes of the ſeaſons, or of heat and cold. In that very different ſpecies, the gangrenous angina, the ancient authors are nearly barren of information: ſome years this is epidemick and contagious in different parts of our iſland; and is much more inimical to childhood and adoleſcence than to adults; diſcharging its venom on ſchools, and the younger branches of families.

The principal differences in inflammatory angina are in the parts affected, and the degrees of inflammation; which may be in one or in both ſides; and variouſly extended over the mucous membrane of the fauces, tonſils, velum, uvula, pharynx, and larynx. The uſual ſymptoms are, local pain and inflammation; more or leſs difficulty of deglutition, reſpiration, and articulation, with clammy exſcreation. The criſis is in a few days; at the utmoſt in a week or

two,

two, by reſolution, or by ſuppuration; ſeldom or ever by gangrene. Suppuration may be artificially diſcharged, or may ſpontaneouſly burſt internally or externally. With judicious and opportune aſſiſtance, there is trifling danger. When fatal, it is by ſuffocation.

The prediſpoſing and occaſional cauſes of angina are, cold air inſpired, cold and moiſt air; perſpiration ſuddenly checked, eſpecially on the neck; cold water drank when the body is heated; epidemical influence of the air and ſeaſons; venereal ſalivation.

Inflammation principally attached to the muſcles of the os hyoides, glottis, larynx, and trachea, or to the tongue, is fortunately far leſs frequent than the former. As in thoſe ſpecies it is obvious there muſt be greater danger of ſtrangulation.

The genorick features of angina gangrenoſa are, ſymptoms of nervous and putrid fever, with ſome inflammation of the fauces and palate of a crimſon colour; ſloughs and ulcerations on tonſils, and ſome difficulty in deglutition. In moſt caſes there is alſo a cutaneous efflореſcence overſpreading variouſly the face, neck, and other parts of the body. This is infinitely more dangerous than the inflammatory angina; terminating ſalutary or fatal from the third to the ſeventh day, according to the degrees of virulence and medical aid. The inauſpicious ſymptoms of debility, putridity, and gangrene, may be gathered from febrile prognoſticks in general. But by the ſpeedy and judicious aſſiſtance of remedies and regimen, very few, compared to the ſick and infected, ſink. It is epidemick and contagious; but of the ſource or nature of the contagion we are unacquainted.

Inflammation of the Lungs and Organs of Reſpiration. I apprehend, that in the London regiſters the mortality by pulmonick inflammation is under-rated, and perhaps delegated to impoſthume and conſumption. This is a frequent inflammation in northern climates; and moſt ſo in ſpring, autumn, and winter; when the body, hydraulick canals, and blood, are in a ſtate of inflammatory diatheſis: it generally encounters the robuſt vigorous conſtitution, thoſe of ſtrong muſcular fibre, and denſe rich blood; the athletick ruſtick, manufacturer, and artizan; thoſe in the prime, and in all the intervals between twenty and the decline of life: it is very rare in infancy, as an idiopathick diſeaſe, and is ſeldom prevalent under puberty, or in old age. It is moſt univerſal amongſt the male ſex; and in all probability, both more univerſal and deſtructive amongſt the neceſſitous laborious maſs of the community. We alſo read in authors, of ſpring pleuriſies as no unuſual affliction in ſome climates conſiderably nearer to the equator than ours.

The primary ſeat of pulmonick inflammation, whether in the parenchyma or internal viſcus, or in its inveſting membranes, is not clearly eſtabliſhed in medical diagnoſticks, and therefore we comprehend pleuriſy and peripneumony under one genus: in moſt caſes they are complicated, and it is now doubted, whether any peripneumony occurs without the pleura alſo participating in the affliction. The ſymptoms of pulmonick inflammation are the general

general precurſors of fever, with darting pungent pain fixed like a dagger in ſome part of the thorax, the ſide, breaſt, or back, and exaſperated by frequent coughing: ſometimes the pain is more dull and obtuſe, and is commonly confined to one lobe: there is alſo load and oppreſſion at the breaſt, accelerated laborious reſpiration, reſtleſſneſs, anxiety. A criſis, when favourable, always enſues between ſeven and fourteen days: generally by expectoration; ſometimes by the other excretories. The termination of pulmonick inflammation is by reſolution, by ſuppuration, by gangrene, by fatal effuſion of blood, or exudation of coagulable lymph into the cellular texture, bronchial verſicles and air pipes; and this, more frequently than gangrene, is the cauſe of ſuffocation and death. The occurrence of either is ſeldom later than a fortnight.

Inauſpicious ſymptoms are, the reſpiration ſtruggling and laborious in the extreme; dry pertinacious cough; no expectoration, or with difficulty; ſuppreſſed expectoration; obtuſe pain, with difficult reſpiration; frequent violent cough exaſperating the pain; the pain changing from one ſide into the other, or continuing immoveable and not diſperſing; the pulmonick lobes in both ſides inflamed; the breathing intolerable and ſuffocating, except in an erect poſture, and even then with laborious anxiety; the face turgid and florid, or pale, with features of conſternation; violent head-ach; delirium; remiſſion ſucceeded by relapſe; exceſſive ſweats; dry ſkin; weak, ſoft, and irregular pulſe; ſudden ceſſation of pain; grumous livid expectoration; rattling noiſe in the thorax, as if plugged up by phlegm;

dejected

dejected countenance, ſqualid ſunk eyes; great proſtration of ſtrength; cold clammy partial ſweats; limpid urine; florid blood coughed up, or white and glutinous matter, reſembling the branches of blood-veſſels. There is alſo great danger of pulmonick inflammation, perſevering beyond ſeven, or, at the utmoſt, fourteen days, and without any conſiderable remiſſion, or ſigns of reſolution, terminating in ſuppuration. Authors have likewiſe deſcribed a malignant peripneumony, which ſeems to be a complication of the preceding deleterious ſymptoms, and of putrid fever.

There is, however, a ſpecies of pulmonick affliction, which is named Peripneumonia Notha; whoſe ſymptoms, at the onſet, are ambiguous: and are, great difficulty in reſpiration; but without concomitant heat or fever. It is moſt frequent in perſons old, phlegmatick, fat, weak, emaciated, ſubject to catarrh, addicted to fermented and ſpirituous liquors. It appears in the ſame ſeaſons with genuine pulmonick inflammation, and with catarrh; that is, in ſpring and autumn; and in foggy and rainy winters; and frequently under the veil of a violent catarrh: and ſometimes ſuddenly and unexpectedly aggravated, ſuffocates the patient.

The prediſpoſing and occaſional cauſes of pulmonick inflammation are, epidemick ſtate of the air; ſudden viciſſitudes of the ſeaſons and weather from heat to cold; ſudden ſuppreſſion of perſpiration, or of pulmonary exhalation; inſpiration of cold air; ſudden expoſure to keen cold air, eſpecially after breathing in a warm room, or drinking warm liquors; cold liquors drank when the body is heated; intemperance and sottishness, particularly in spirituous liquors; dry cold winds; strong muscular exercise, or manual labour; repulsion of cutaneous eruption, febrile or chronic; exsiccation of old ulcers; suppression of habitual evacuation and eruption; translation to and deposition of morbid matter on the lungs; consequence and dregs of small-pox and measles; symptomatick from some other diseases.

Inflammations of the Heart, Mediastinum and Diaphragm, as solitary, are very rare diseases. The physiology and pathology of these organs will naturally lead to the discrimination of their inflammation. When paraphrenitis occurs, it is generally complicated with inflammation of the adjacent organs in either the thorax or abdomen. As the heart is the main spring of the blood's circulation, and the diaphragm the principal agent in respiration, it is evident that inflammation in either must be extremely dangerous.

Inflammation of the Liver, hepatitis, acute and chronic. Both species are much more frequent in tropical climates and warm regions, than in northern and cold; and more so in the former, during the hottest seasons of the year. The sensibility of the liver being dull, its inflammation is less painful than that of any other viscus. It invades with obtuse pain, heat, and heaviness in the hepatick region; with some fever; generally with a jaundice tinge of the eyes, countenance, and urine, and with increased discharge of bile. But the different parts of the liver inflamed, or its complication with that of the adjacent

jacent organs, will diverſify the ſymptoms. The acute hepatitis, but not the chronic, is uſually terminated in a few days, at the utmoſt fourteen or twenty-one, by diſcuſſion and evacuation of bile through ſome of the larger excretories; and by ſuppuration; and by gangrene. Suppuration is not an unfrequent termination: after which many ſurvive, but with difficult and ſlow recovery. The purulency may be variouſly expurgated by abſorption, by the biliary ducts, by eroſion of the abdominal muſcles, or by an artificial opening when the abſceſs is perceptible externally; and ſometimes it erodes the diaphragm and lungs.

The prediſpoſing and occaſional cauſes of hepatitis are, burning climates; acrid viſcid bile; the blood tenacious and glutinous in conſiſtence; calculi, ſteatome, worms in the biliary ducts; bilious vomiting; ſudden refrigeration of the body when heated, and obſtructed perſpiration; thirſt, and not ſufficient dilution of the blood; intoxication and abuſe of ſpirituous liquors; poiſons; external injuries; violent exerciſe; paſſions of mind; inveterate hypochondriaſm; tranſlation of purulent matter to the liver; ſymptomatick.

Inflammation of the Stomach, gaſtritis. Notwithſtanding the inceſſant irritation and diſtention of this ſenſible organ, by innumerable varieties of food and drink, yet its inflammation is a rare event. The ſymptoms are, fixed burning pain and heat, nauſea, vomiting, reſtleſſneſs, univerſal debility. It may prove fatal in the ſpace of a few days, or even of a few hours: there are different gradations of ſeverity and danger.

danger. The termination is by refolution, fuppuration, gangrene.

The predifpofing and occafional caufes of gaftritis are, all the caufes of topical inflammations in general; poifons fwallowed; cold water, ices, and fruits fwallowed when the body is much heated; repletion from food and gormandizing; crude and difficultly digefted nutriment; violent agitation of body or mind; external injuries: repelled gout very rarely.

Eryfipelas, ignis fanct. antonii: gutta rofacea, zofter, zona, herpes. Some trifling pillage by this local cutaneous inflammation is noticed in the London bills. It varioufly affails the furface of the face, the neck, the trunk, or one of the extremities with pain, rednefs, tenfion, and pruriency; and is moft hoftile to adults. It is fometimes critical and falutary: the favourable crifis is ufually in a few days, or within nine, by perfpiration, urine, and defquamation of the inflamed cuticle; and fometimes without any perceptible revulfion to the excretories: never by fuppuration. Some have this cutaneous inflammation annually, or oftener, or at wider intervals; and thofe once affected, are more obnoxious to its returns. Prefages of danger are, violent inflammation and intumefcence, efpecially on the face, or fometimes even on the legs, and particularly in old age, or unfound conftitutions; premature retroceffion of the eruption; pale colour; frequent return, and repetition of the inflammation; delirium; coma; gangrene. On the legs it fometimes leaves behind a chronic enlargement.

The

The predispoſing and occaſional cauſes of Eryſipelas are, epidemick influence of the air; obſtructed perſpiration; ſudden refrigeration of the body when heated; plethora; ſuppreſſed evacuations, natural or artificial; luxurious living and indolence; intemperance; ſpirituous liquors in exceſs; poiſons; unſound conſtitutions; contuſions, wounds, burns, punctured nerves, bliſters, acrids; dregs of fevers; ſcorbutick; lunar influence; paſſions of mind.

Rheumatiſm, acute and chronic. From the Chart of diſeaſes we may rank rheumatiſm rather as a ſcourge and inſtrument of torture than of execution. In the acute or chronic form, multitudes are moleſted by it, eſpecially in this iſland, and in northern regions: and more ſo in winter, ſpring, and autumn, and the interchanges of the ſeaſons: it ſeldom moleſts very young or aged perſons: adults are moſt annoyed by it; the male more than the female ſex; the poor and indigent more than the affluent; and thoſe moſt who are expoſed to the inclemency and viciſſitudes of the ſeaſons and weather: hence, during war, ſoldiers and ſailors are much more afflicted with it than in peace.

In the acute rheumatiſm, the fever may commence before or after the pain, which variouſly and alternately ſeems to dilacerate different parts, eſpecially about the joints of the ancles, knees, hips, ſhoulders, elbows, and wriſts, ſometimes the trunk, but rarely the ſmall joints of the toes or fingers; and commonly ſucceeded by ſwelling and redneſs of the diſtracted joints, and with reſtleſſneſs: at night the pains are exaſperated, and often ſuddenly abating in one joint, ſeize

ſeize upon another; thus harraſſing the body with a war of poſts. Its continuance may be one, two, or three weeks; by which time the fever, if not miſmanaged, abates with the pains: it very rarely terminates in ſuppuration, and in this inſtance reſembles eryſipelas and gout. It may terminate inauſpiciouſly in chronic pains, or in conſumption: indeed, emaciation is always a conſequence.

Chronic rheumatiſm without fever or inflammation, but often with direful pain and torture, and often with extreme difficulty or inability to perform muſcular motion, may occupy all the ſtations of the acute: in the hips it is called iſchias, morbus coxendicis, and ſciatica; in the loins, lumbago. The latter of theſe, from ignorance in morbid diagnoſticks, may be confounded with nephritis; and it may ſo happen, fatally for the patient. Chronic rheumatiſm may harraſs months, years, with various degrees of ſeverity and exacerbation, and interludes of eaſe; and is often extremely obſtinate and difficult to be diſlodged. In many inſtances alſo, we obſerve a contrariety and dilemma, whether to affix the name of chronic rheumatiſm or gout to ſuch pains. But in general, rheumatick aches are not ſo periodical in their returns; and in ſeveral other features the two diſeaſes divaricate.

The prediſpoſing and occaſional cauſes of acute and chronic rheumatiſm, idiopathick and ſymptomatick, are, ſudden ſuppreſſion of perſpiration; ſudden heats and colds; cold damp night air, beds, houſes, habitations, want of ſufficient warm cloathing and fuel in rigorous ſeaſons, or during the interchanges of the ſeaſons; wet cloaths;

cloaths; expoſure to heats and colds; ſudden viciſſitudes of heat and cold; change of winds and weather; one part of the body expoſed to cold whilſt the other part is heated; ſleeping on damp ground; plethora; impure blood; repelled eruption; ſuppreſſed evacuations; habitual intoxication; intermittent; dregs of fever, arthritick; hereditary; ſcorbutick; hyſterical: venereal; noxious exhalation from lead or mercury; exceſs of venery; tabes dorſalis; aneuriſm of the deſcending aorta near the loins; lifting great weights; internal abſceſs and ſcirrhus; abſceſs, and caries at the upper articulation of the thigh-bone; ſprains; luxation and fracture of its neck; diſeaſes of the coverings of the nerves, or of their medullary ſubſtance, or of the muſcular fibre.

Gout, arthritis, podagra; acute, chronic, regular, and irregular. In the preceding century it was confounded with ſciatica in the London bills. During the preſent century, there is a conſiderable increaſe in the arthritick mortality: but, compared to ſome other of the morbid hoſt, it is a petty foe. Arthritick mortality muſt ſolely be imputed to the aſſaults of chronic gout, either gradually breaking down the fabrick, or ſuddenly ſtorming ſome of the internal organs eſſential to life. Compared to the number afflicted, very few die of this diſeaſe. It has even been by ſome conſidered as an omen of longevity: many ſubject to it have reached the Moſaick goal. It has alſo been alledged, to render men more ſecure from other diſeaſes, and in ſome few inſtances to expurgate and renovate a diſordered conſtitution. Theſe obſer-

vations,

vations, however, muſt be reſtricted to regular gout only, and recurring at diſtant intervals.

Here we have no foundation to accuſe the elements, or the inviſible demons of diſeaſe. This malady, either immediately or by hereditary deſcent, is too often the natural caſtigation and penance of voluptuouſneſs and ſenſuality. The gout attacks principally the male ſex; ſometimes, but rarely, females; and of the latter thoſe of robuſt full habits, the viragines, luxurious, indolent, corpulent, and generally after the final menſtrual ceſſation: the majority, from the peculiarity in the female conſtitution, and from ſuperiority in temperance, are exempt. It ſeldom attacks before middle age; generally in the decline of life: the few exceptions of its earlier occurrence are rare; and in them it is uſually by co-operation of hereditary, and of remote exciting cauſes: in adoleſcence, and before puberty, it would be numbered amongſt the medical miracles. It haraſſes moſt thoſe of robuſt, full, corpulent, large frame, and temperament, the voracious, gormandizing, affluent, and pampered; more of the patrician than the plebeian orders; more of the literary and ſedentary profeſſions; and, according to Sydenham, thoſe of an acute genius and intellectual eminence. The active and induſtrious orders of every community; thoſe who are exerciſed in daily corporeal labour, or who, from neceſſity, deſign, cuſtom, or religion, do not indulge to exceſs in animal food, or in wine and fermented liquors, are ſeldom arthritick martyrs.

That periodical local pain and inflammation, called the regular arthritick paroxiſm, ſometimes invades ſuddenly, without any warning; but in general there are preſages of its approach, indicated by ſome unuſual diſorder of the animal ſpirits, of the muſcular energy, and of the digeſtive organs. The regular and recent paroxiſm commonly invades by nocturnal ſurprize in bed, with excruciating pain in one foot, uſually the ball of the great toe, accompanied with ſhivering, heat, and ſhortly after, conſpicuous gloſſy redneſs, tenſion, and ſpreading tumor. In this way there are more or leſs diurnal remiſſions and exacerbations of pain; which, after one, two, three, or four weeks, recedes gradually and inſenſibly, together with the redneſs and ſwelling; leaving the patient, who had been chained to a bed or couch, in perfect health; and ſoon after, the foot in the exerciſe of its former ſuppleneſs and ſtrength.

At the beginning of the diſeaſe the pain is more ſevere, the paroxiſms are ſhorter, and the periods more regular and diſtant; at intervals of three or four years, or longer: by degrees the intervals are progreſſively reduced to two years, to one year; to two paroxiſms annually about the equinoxes and ſolſtices, and during the autumn, winter, and ſpring; at the ſame time the paroxiſms are protracted to two or three months. At length, in the chronic inveterate ſtages of the diſeaſe the patient enjoys a very ſhort reſpite; ſome few of the enervated, perhaps only two or three months during the ſummer: the pains in the extremities are then indeed leſs violent, but the ſtomach is more diſordered. In recent gout, one foot only is aſſaulted; by degrees both feet, one after the other;

other: and in the rooted ſtate of the diſeaſe it not only torments both feet in ſucceſſion, but capriciouſly deſerts and re-attacks various parts; the ancle, knee, elbow, wriſt; darting often with electrical velocity and ſhocks through the nerves and muſcular fibres: thus, in a circle of torture and litigious warfare, teazing the arthritick victim.

When either the inflammation of the joints has commenced in the uſual manner, but without an adequate degree of pain and inflammation, or at leaſt without continuing the uſual time, and pecipitately recedes, ſome internal organ is expoſed in its retreat and rebound. Or when the arthritick fuel is occluded, and not ejected to the feet, eſpecially at the uſual periods, it will, according to the various parts and organs affected, excite correſponding vibrations and morbid ſymptoms in the natural, vital, and animal functions; as inappetency, indigeſtion, nauſea, vomiting, flatulence, eructation, colick, diarrhœa, nephritis, and urinary obſtructions; difficult reſpiration, aſthma, palpitation, fainting, general debility, low ſpirits, hypochondriaſm, muſcular ſpaſms, head-ach, apoplexy, palſy: and it is of the higheſt moment to know that theſe numerous morbid ſymptoms are rarely of an inflammatory nature. After the diſeaſe has continued many years with frequent reiterated paroxiſms the joints do not ſoon recover, but continue weak and ſtiff. In many caſes, chalky and calculous concretions are formed in the articulations of the extremities, and in the kidneys and urinary paſſages. Racked by theſe combined tortures, the arthritick martyr requires the auxiliary aid of ſtuffed chairs, flannel, and crutches. The prognoſticks of cure in this ſtage, are conciſely expreſſed in the following lines of one of our native poets, Fenton, and addreſſed to the gout:

Thou that do'ſt Eſculapius deride,
And o'er his gallipots in triumph ride,
Begot on Venus, by the god of wine, &c.

The prediſpoſing and occaſional cauſes of gout are hereditary; inactive ſedentary life, with luxurious living and gormandizing, eſpecially on animal food; intemperance in wine, ſpirituous or fermented liquors; early or intemperate libations to Bacchus and Venus; unremitting application to ſtudy or buſineſs; ſedentary life; nocturnal lucubrations; diſturbed ſleep, cares, misfortunes, vexation, depreſſing paſſions; ceaſing of uſual exerciſe or labour; ſudden tranſition from an active to a ſedentary life; coaches, diſſipation, luxury, effeminacy; ſudden violent changes in diet; plethora; ſuppreſſed evacuations; profuſe evacuations; various cauſes of debility; indigeſtion from quantity or quality of aliment.

Of internal Suppuration in the lungs, liver, ſtomach, inteſtines, kidneys. Pulmonick ſuppuration, empyema, or vomica, may be predicted from preceding inflammation, without conſiderable remiſſions, the neglect of effectual remedies, and no ſigns of reſolution by the efforts of nature or art, and by remiſſion of acute pain; the difficulty of reſpiration, and the cough continuing; with the additional uſual ſymptoms

of

of internal formation of pus; which are frequent horrors and chillineſs, heat and hectic, weight and throbbing in the ſide, thirſt, fetid breath, emaciation. It may burſt in all the intervals between fourteen and ſixty days, and either relieves or ſuffocates, or is gradually expectorated, or expurgated by ſome emunctory, or diſcharged internally. Sometimes there are ſeveral ſmall abſceſſes; and too frequently the final termination is ulceration and phthiſis. Suppuration in the liver is a frequent conſequence of previous inflammation, and is not altogether ſo fatal as ſome other internal abſceſſes. Its ſymptoms are thoſe in common with internal formation of pus, and accompanied with a jaundice colour of the eyes. Sometimes the purulence erodes the external integuments; or the diaphragm, lungs, or ſtomach; ſometimes it is diſcharged by the biliary ducts into the inteſtines, or abſorbed and waſhed away with the urine. Suppuration in the ſtomach and inteſtines is very rare. Suppuration in the kidneys is accompanied with the general ſymptoms, and with purulent fetid urine: it may alſo burſt externally; or by ſlow ulceration and hectic, undermine the conſtitution.

Of *Internal Gangrene* in the lungs, ſtomach, nteſtines, kidneys, liver. Pulmonick gangrene rom inflammation, is predicted by ſudden ceſation of pain, without any benign criſis; by expectoration, either ſuppreſſed, or yellow, green, black, and fetid; by hollow noiſe in the breaſt during reſpiration; dejected countenance; red and heavy eyes; foul and black tongue; quick, languid, and intermittent pulſe; fetid urine, feces, and ſweat; hiccup; cold ſweats; univerſal debility and ſinking of the vital powers. From the preceding ſymptoms, from thoſe enumerated under general febrile prognoſticks, and from the functions peculiar to the different diſeaſed organs, internal gangrene in whatſoever part may be comprehended; and a minute detail would be ſurperfluous.

CHAP VI.

DISEASES of the Lungs and Organs of Reſpiration, what extenſive ruin do they yet ſpread! Inflammation of theſe organs and ſpurious peripneumony, have already been deſcribed. Theſe, therefore, together with the preſent group, conſtitute nearly the whole combined pulmonick hoſt, and likewiſe ſome of thoſe diſeaſes cloſely connected with the pneumonick machinery, or with ſeveral of its general morbid ſymptoms. Behold here one of the great caravans of dead to the ſtygian ferry; and tottering myriads crowding to the ſame ſhambles. Every introſpection of morbid regiſters, and the unanimous obſervations of the medical profeſſion, concord in proclaiming the notoriety of the conſumptive throng, and their ruinous domination. Notwithſtanding the immenſe improvement in the alphabet, ſubordinate rudiments,

diments, and appendages of the medical ſcience, conſumption as yet is one of the oligarchy of morbid and remorſeleſs tyrants.

From one *fifth* to one *ſixth* of all the mortality in London, is from conſumption; which is nearly double to that even of ſmall-pox. But conſumption is a term too lax and indefinite. Into this gulph, no doubt, are thrown many febrile and ſlow hectick emaciations, from infancy to old age, in both ſexes; and there are few diſeaſes from acute and chronic ſources, eſpecially in their fatal termination, without emaciation and cachexy. Conſumptions and dropſies are the final wreck of a prodigious variety of human maladies. In no two other diſeaſes are, what pathologiſts term *Morbi a Morbis*, more apparent; and in multitudes of ſuch caſes, morbid diſſections often detect the effect, and not the original cauſe. How many of the genuine pulmonary phthiſis are conſociated with this miſcellaneous crowd, is difficult to gueſs; but, from the concurrent teſtimony of phyſicians, and of experience, we may ſafely affirm a very large proportion. There are few families in this kingdom whom it has not, one time or other, plunged into tears. Phyſicians on the continent alledge, that phthiſis is more prevalent in Britain than in any other kingdom of Europe: and many of them alledge it to be contagious.

The next inquiry is, in what age, ſex, rank of life, ſeaſon of the year, and whether in city or country is conſumption moſt predominant? It has been, from the earlieſt chronology, the univerſal echo and monotony of medical writers, to mark the principal conſumptive age between 18 and 35. But, with ſubmiſſion, I would conſiderably enlarge its limits, including from birth to 5, and from 20 to 60. No age or ſtage of life is exempted; but we might "*a priori*," and from viewing the great and general ſcale of mortality, aſſert, that between 5 and 20, a conſiderable number cannot poſſibly be ſwept away in the phthiſical torrent. Nor do we mean to invalidate the general aphoriſm, that in the bloſſom and full maturity of vigour and comelineſs, phthiſis is ſuperlatively deleterious. Between the ſexes no diſtinction ſeems to be made. I conceive, however, that amongſt the lower orders univerſally, and more eſpecially thoſe penned up in the foul atmoſphere of cities, that phthiſis is more fatal than amongſt thoſe who browſe in the pure air of the country. In accommodation, cloathing, noxious trades, &c. the indigent have alſo the diſadvantage; and during ſickneſs, from the ſame cauſes, their recovery is more deſperate. With reſpect to ſeaſons, winter and autumn in our climate is the moſt pernicious to pulmonick maladies,

Pulmonary Hemorrhage, hæmoptyſis, ſputum ſanguinis. The lungs ſpungy pneumatick and hydraulick organs, are in themſelves paſſive: but by the contraction of the diaphragm and intercoſtal muſcles enlarging the capacity of the thorax, this ventilator is alternately diſtended with atmoſpheric air, and this ſonorous fluid again quickly expelled, with either ſome noxious emanation from the body, or decompoſition of its own vital principle. Half the blood of the human body circulates through this organ:

gan; its blood-veſſels are numerous and large, and riſe immediately from the heart; and it is inceſſantly in motion and agitation.

When the body has nearly attained its ultimate extenſion and altitude, Pulmonary hemorrhage is moſt predominant; more eſpecially in thoſe of narrow thorax, prominent ſcapulæ, red cheeks, and acute tone of voice. It is manifeſted by cough, exſpuition of florid blood in various quantity, and ſlowly or ſuddenly, from ounces to pounds, or even quarts, in a few days; but the latter is rare. It may ſoon totally ceaſe, or only intermit, and again return at irregular intervals. Relapſes are frequent on any irregularity or intemperance; on acceleration of the circulation, or expanſion from heat. This hemorrhage is very ſeldom in ſuch quantities as to prove precipitately fatal, unleſs miſmanaged. From bleeding, at leaſt in the London regiſters, there is petty ſpoliation. Pulmonary hemorrhage is more frequently the conſumptive precurſor. Malign omens are an eruptive torrent; ulceration in the lungs; fever renewed; pain in the breaſt; difficulty of breathing; cough, hoarſeneſs; night ſweats; peripneumony; viſceral obſtructions; cachexy; old age; relapſes. But pulmonary hemorrhage from temporary obſtructions of the menſes, or in pregnancy, or periodical, or without load in the thorax, or fever, are much leſs miſchievous.

Pulmonary Phthiſis. Not one hundredth part of pulmonary conſumptions commence with hemorrhage. The phthiſical lineaments are emaciation, diurnal hectic fever, obſtinate rebellious cough, difficulty of breathing, and uſually ſome change

change in the voice. In the beginning, phthisis often resembles a catarrh, or stubborn cold; and in this insidious disguise is too frequently slighted, or neglected: but continuing longer than the usual catarrhal period, without any considerable intermission, and especially if in summer, are sufficient grounds to alarm. In that, from tubercles, there is frequent teazing dry cough, exasperated at night; some difficulty of breathing, and panting on ascending any eminence or stairs, or on exercise; some emaciation and weakness. By degrees, there is more or less expectoration of viscid, yellow, greenish purulence, intermixed, however, with natural mucus, and in the progress often streaked with blood: and sooner or later, uneasiness in the breast. The cough and expectoration in frequency and quantity, consistence and colour, vary in different persons. The consuming hectic has generally two exacerbations during the twenty-four hours, about noon and night; with some degree of chilliness and shivering, and increased sensibility to cool air, notwithstanding the skin and palms of the hands are preternaturally hot.

In this island, phthisis, especially from tubercles not suppurated, may continue one, two, or more years; appearing during the winter and spring, and disappearing during the summer. Other consumptions are much more rapid; in the vernacular phrase, galloping the patient to a skeleton in a few months. Phthisical patients are rarely confined to bed, until near the deplorable stages and fatal termination. Some have even a tolerable appetite; and the generality

generality are cheered with adulatory hopes of recovery to the laſt extremity. The progreſſive encroachment of the diſeaſe is evident, by increaſed debility, emaciation, and partial ſweats; edematous ancles; diarrhœa; depilation; conſumption and melting away of the fat and muſcular fleſh: until at laſt ſapleſs, and macerated into ghoſts, the twinkling vital ſnuff is extinguiſhed.

It is, as yet, impoſſible for me to apportion the comparative mortality and recovery in real confirmed phthiſis; nor could I depend upon any of the general regiſters which I carefully conſulted with this view. We may, however, venture upon a groſs eſtimate, by negative proof. Excluſive of individual evidence, and medical atteſtation, we might, by a ſimple algebraic proceſs out of any ſpecified number, with their mortal diſeaſes, and probable proportion of ſick in each, ſift out the conſumptive. At all events, it cannot poſſibly be thought exaggeration to alledge, that under the preſent imperfect practice, a very conſiderable majority of the conſumptive die. From hereditary entail or tubercles it is ſtill more deſperate. But, on the other hand, the mortality, notoriouſly, by conſumption, and indeed in all other diſeaſes, will be prodigiouſly varied by an early or too late application to ſkilful advice.

Species of Conſumption are, hectic fever, atrophy and tabes; nervous; icterick; dorſal. Hectick fever and atrophy is deſcribed as a very frequent and fatal diſeaſe of infants, eſpecially in cities; accompanied with emaciation, often with ſhort dry cough, with hot ſkin and palms of the hands; with quick pulſe, thirſt, diurnal exacerbations, ſickly countenance: in ſome the abdomen is alſo tumid, and conſiderably enlarged. Atrophy and Nervous tabes are confounded in medical diagnoſticks: in both there is emaciation; but no conſiderable fever, cough, or difficulty of breathing; but impaired appetite and digeſtion, and ſometimes morbid voraciouſneſs; leucophlegmatick ſickly appearance, partial ſweats; general debility, and proneneſs to faint on any exertion. The icterick tabes is accompanied with ſymptoms of jaundice; and probably, under ſeveral diſguiſes, is more frequent than medical authors have repreſented. In ſome of the quadruped race it is a very univerſal cauſe of cachexy, rot and mortality.

Dorſal, or ſpermatick conſumption is a particular ſpecies; miſerable ſpectacles of which are recorded by the celebrated Tiſſot. It is diſtinguiſhed by nocturnal involuntary pollution, and debility in the nervous and muſcular energy. By degrees, the appetite decays with indigeſtion, hypochondriaſm, melancholy; with pains in various parts, head-ach, lumbago, univerſal debility, waſting of the penis, impotency and blight of future progeny. Females are not exempt from this diſeaſe; but it is much more frequent amongſt the male ſex, and from the age of puberty through various adult ſtages of life. The foundation of it is often laid at ſchools; and in thoſe ſeminaries of vice, large cities: and in ſome countries it is a more general habit of licentiouſneſs than in others.

Of the prediſpoſing and occaſional cauſes of pulmonary hemorrhage, pulmonary phthiſis,

hectick,

hectick, atrophy and tabes. Of pulmonary hemorrhage; hereditary; narrow thorax; weak pulmonary blood veſſels, ſmall capacity; plethora; ſuppreſſion of natural or habitual hemorrhage, as naſal, hemorrhoidal, menſtrual; amputation of a conſiderable extremity; luxurious living and indolence; violent exertion and exerciſe of the lungs and voice in various trades and profeſſions; alſo violent efforts to cough, to exonerate the excretories, parturition; lifting great weights; violent exerciſe; furious paſſions of mind: external injuries on the thorax; wounds; confinement of the thorax by writing-deſks, by ſtrong whalebone ſtays; ſuppreſſed perſpiration and exhalation of the ſkin and lungs by cold; light atmoſphere, eſpecially on high mountains; pulmonick inflammation; ſcrophulous lymphatick glands and tubercles in the lungs, or calculous concretions; polypus concretions in the large pulmonary blood-veſſels; ſchirrus and obſtruction in the abdominal viſcera.

The prediſpoſing and occaſional cauſes of pulmonary phthiſis are all the preceding cauſes of pulmonick hemorrhage; hereditary; ſcrophulous tubercles; ſuppuration in the lungs, and not with laudable pus; calculi in the lungs; conſequence of pulmonick inflammation and ſuppuration, of ſmall-pox, meaſles; hooping cough, rickets, and of various acute and chronic diſeaſes; venereal, icterick; chloroſis; worms; rheumatiſm; chronic aſthma; internal abſceſſes and ulcers; catarrh and neglected colds; ſudden ſuppreſſion of perſpiration, eſpecially when the body is heated; ſuppreſſion of pulmonary exhalation

halation, and inſpiration of cold damp air; irregularity and coldneſs of the climate joined to moiſture; various noxious trades and occupations; inſpiration of noxious fumes and effluvia; foul atmoſphere of cities, coal fires; broken ribs, and blows on the thorax; indigence; cold habitations; inſufficient cloathing and fuel in rigorous ſeaſons.

The prediſpoſing and occaſional cauſes of hectic, atrophy and tabes, are many of the cauſes juſt now enumerated; ſcrophulous obſtructed meſenterick glands, and courſe of the chyle; colds; damp habitations; foul atmoſphere of cities; moiſt cloudy atmoſphere; unwholeſome air; coagulated milk in the ſtomach and inteſtines; foul ſtomach; diſeaſed ſtomach and abdominal viſcera; improper diet; gluttony, ſloth, uncleanlineſs, bad nurſing, inſufficient exerciſe; worms; repelled cutaneous eruptions and ulcers; cachexy; intoxication and intemperance; depreſſing paſſions of mind, cares, and vexations; intenſe ſtudy; inſufficient nutriment, poverty, and want of food; frequent vomiting of food; faults in the organs of digeſtion; defect or depravity of the digeſtive fluids, profuſe evacuations, as hemorrhages, diarrhœa, diäbetes, fluor albus, ſalivation, ſeminal emiſſion; delicate women ſuckling; ſweats; rupture of the thoracick duct; diſeaſes of the ſpinal brain; weakneſs of the ſolidum vivum; general defect of fluids, or of oil in the cellular texture; fever and abſorption of the ſubcutaneous oil; old age and contraction of the ſmall veſſels; broken conſtitution, from various cauſes; frequent manuſtupration; libidinous books, prints; conſe-

quence

quence of venereal gleets, and improper treatment.

Aſthma. In the London bills, aſthma and tiſſick are incorporated: formerly it was conſumption and tiſſick, the Italian name for conſumption, and without any mention of aſthma. It would appear by the London regiſters, that about one *fortieth part* of the funerals is from aſthma; and its proportion to conſumptive mortality as 1 to 8. I have every reaſon to believe that the funeral catalogue in London is not, in any outrageous degree, overcharged with conſumption or aſthma. As both theſe diſeaſes are properly excluded from in-patients of our hoſpitals, I applied to one of the largeſt diſpenſaries in London, the Alderſgate; in which there is neceſſarily an overflow of both theſe diſtempers; and with the intention of confronting and irradiating the bills of mortality. Almoſt every page of theſe books preſented aſthma in no inconſiderable number; but above all, phthiſis, phthiſis, towering with gigantic bulk.

A TABLE, demonſtrating the comparative proportion of aſthma and dyſpnœa to other diſeaſes in London; the proportion of males and females afflicted with this diſeaſe; the ages or ſtages of life when aſthma is moſt predominant; the proportion of cured, relieved, diſcharged, and dead in this diſeaſe; founded upon the regiſters of the Alderſgate Diſpenſary, from 1770 to 1788.

Of 70,000 patients, aſthma and dyſpnœa were 3,192: aſthmatick males, 1613; aſthmatick

tick females 1536. The ſundry ages of theſe aſthmaticks were:

Comparative ages.		*Numbers.*
From birth to 10 years	—	36
10 to 20	——	25
20 to 30	——	161
30 to 40	——	429
40 to 50	——	882
50 to 60	——	949
60 to 70 and upwards		710

Cured.		*Relieved.*		*Diſcharged.*		*Dead.*
1879	—	575	——	569	—	169

From the preceding valuable records we may draw the following inferences: that aſthma and dyſpnœa conſtitute, at leaſt in that diſpenſary, the proportion of 1 to 22 of the diſeaſes: that it is ſomewhat more predominant in the male than the female ſex: that in infancy and adoleſcence there are very few caſes of aſthma and dyſpnœa: that theſe diſeaſes chiefly occur in middle age and the decline of life: that more than one half of them are reported as cured; the relieved and diſcharged forming a neutral liſt, numbers of whom were either ſurfeited with medicines, or were diſcharged by their phyſicians when deſpairing of a radical cure, or fearful of their ſwelling the dead catalogue: in ſinking of which there is a univerſal rivalſhip throughout our diſpenſaries and hoſpitals. Some of them, probably, were palliated; and indeed many were labouring with age, for whom it would be unreaſonable to expect a radical cure. I conceive, that with a part of them we may venture to double the dead liſt; which would raiſe

raiſe aſthmatick mortality to one of ten. But in the above eſtimate, what proportion legitimate periodick aſthma bears to the other anhelations I could not fathom.

The term aſthma has been miſapplied to every ſpecies of dyſpnœa: it ſtrictly denotes a chronic periodic difficulty of breathing, recurring and exaſperated in paroxiſms, ſometimes almoſt to the degree of ſuffocation; and, at leaſt in the intervals, without fever. Authors have ſubdivided it into ſeveral ſpecies; the ſpaſmodic, convulſive, and periodical; the dry, humid, continued, flatulent: and from the gradations of difficulty in reſpiration, into dyſpnœa, orthopnœa. The periodick and ſpaſmodick is the true diſeaſe.

In the duration, recurrence, intermiſſion, and remiſſion, aſthmatic paroxiſms vary. A few hours, or a few days, are the uſual limits of this pulmonick tumult. In the beginning it continues only a few hours, with a diurnal remiſſion and nocturnal renovation: in the chronic ſtate, from two to five days is the uſual duration. The intermiſſions are proportioned to the duration of the paroxiſms: the longer the paroxiſms the longer the intervals, and *vice verſa:* with a copious expectoration they ſooner terminate, and are leſs ſevere. Some have had as many paroxiſms in winter as in ſummer; and in the country as in town. Floyer had ſixty in winter and twenty in ſummer: the latter, as uſual, were more violent, and longer. During calm froſty weather aſthmaticks are more ſecure; but at all points of the compaſs the paroxiſm may invade. Some find more eaſe in the city than country; others, in low ground than mountainous. Some are never entirely liberated from dyſpnœa, and with periodical aggravations. Few, comparatively, die immediately, in the aſthmatick paroxiſms: numbers ſurvive many years, even to the goal of longevity, and emaciation excepted, without conſiderable diminution of ſtrength, ſpirits, or appetite. After long continuance, it ſeldom admits of a radical cure; but only alleviation and reſpite. Its fatal terminations are ſuffocation, apoplexy, pulmonick inflammation, conſumption, cachexy, partial or general dropſy; polypi in the heart and the large veſſels.

The prediſpoſing and occaſional cauſes of aſthma are hereditary; original ſtructure of the pneumonick organs; narrow thorax; plethora; ſuppreſſion of habitual or natural evacuations, and cutaneous eruptions, as menſes, piles, old ulcers, ſweat of the feet; conſequence of catarrh and colds, and ſudden ſuppreſſion of perſpiration: ſerum, pituita in exceſs; cachexy; dregs of fever, ſmall-pox, meaſles, and pulmonick inflammation; pulmonick tubercles; ſpaſmodick ſtricture of the diaphragm and bronchiæ; ſmoky rooms and houſes, eſpecially with wood fires; noxious mineral and metallick fumes, arſenical, nitrous, ſulphureous, ſaturnine; ſmoky atmoſphere of cities; pulverulent trades, as ſtone-cutters, lapidaries, millers, flax-dreſſers, chimney-ſweepers; fetid offenſive ſmells; ſudden changes of weather and winds from heavy to a light atmoſphere, portending ſtorms, and eſpecially ſnow; eaſterly winds; fogs, with unſteadineſs of weather and ſeaſons; poſſibly ſome ſecret alterations in the electrick fluid, and affecting electrometers; warm and moiſt air; errors and intemperance in food and drink, and ingurgitation; violent motion and agitation of body and of mind; ſymptomatick in various diſeaſes, as hyſtericks, hypochondriaſm, gout, pectoral dropſy, empyema, polypi in the heart or aorta; wounds of the lungs; diſeaſes of the liver and ſpleen.

Dyſpnœa and Coughs are ſymptoms of many diſeaſes; and they are alſo primary, and very general maladies, eſpecially in this iſland. It is true, we have here no compaſs to ſteer by: theſe are an exploted banditti; a ſort of rebels againſt the ſymmetry of ſyſtem, whoſe diagnoſticks and theraputicks are as yet ſlovenly and imperfectly noticed by medical authors. From the univerſal connection of the organs of reſpiration, their functions are more or leſs interrupted by and warped with other diſeaſes and morbid ſymptoms. Many of the chronic impediments in breathing, and the broken-winded, may be called aſthmatick excreſcences, without its periodical paroxiſms, exacerbations, and remiſſions; and alſo without any rapid emaciation or hectick: they are ſpurious aſthmas and chronic catarrhs. All the parts about the fauces and pharynx are crowded with mucous glands, from which, as in angina and catarrh, there is often a profuſe ſecretion. Many perſons advanced in life, and the aged, have a large diſcharge of mucus, variouſly, from the fauces, pharynx, larynx, lungs, ſtomach; all requiring frequent expectoration or hawking.

The prediſpoſing and occaſional cauſes of dyſpnœa and coughs are many of thoſe already enumerated under conſumption and aſthma: alſo cold pituitous temperament; air hot, cold, weighty, light, moiſt, impure, ſtagnant; changes and viciſſitudes of the winds; cold moiſt climate and atmoſphere, and eſpecially in winter, autumn, and ſpring, and interchanges of the ſeaſons: ſudden viciſſitudes, diſorders and inconſtancy of the ſurrounding elements; ſuppreſſed perſpiration, and pulmonary exhalation; catarrhal defluxion on the lungs, larynx, fauces; mucus in exceſs, tenacious; faults in the mucus glands and ducts; trachea too ſenſible or irritable; calculi, chalky concretions, and inſpiſſated mucus in the larynx; vaſcular or parenchymatous diſeaſes of the lungs; original faults of the lungs, bronchiæ, larynx; waſted lungs; extravaſated air; ſpaſm of the reſpiratory muſcles; flatulent farinaceous ſlimy food, and drink; weak or foul ſtomach, voraciouſneſs; overflow of ſaliva ſwallowed by infants; ſymptomatick in various diſeaſes of the thorax, as conſumption, aſthma, empyema, polypus, aneuriſm, *cum multis aliis:* ſymptomatick in various diſeaſes of the abdomen interrupting the play of the diaphragm; as full ſtomach, flatulence; pregnancy; dropſy; enlarged ſpleen or liver; tympany; nephritis; worms; injured abdominal muſcles.

Catarrhs, colds, influenza, coryza, gravedo, coughs, hoarſeneſs, rheums, ſternutation, diſtillation from the eyes, noſe, and fauces of acrid lymph; ſoreneſs of the throat and fauces; frequent exſcreation. In our irregular climate, during

during the annual revolution of the ſeaſons, few eſcape ſlight catarrhs and colds, to which all ages are liable. Some catarrhs or colds affect principally the membrane of the noſe, and the different ſinuſſes or cavities communicating with that emunctory: others are lower ſituated in the fauces, pharynx, or trachea. Catarrh ſeldom continues beyond a few days, or weeks: but when it originates from contagion it is more chronic and febrile. That particular epidemick ſpecies of erratick catarrh, called Influenza, has ſometimes ſpread ſuddenly over a kingdom, and over the greateſt part of Europe. In no other epidemick do ſo few die in proportion to the number infected. Its continuance is generally ſhort; and the little depredations committed during its incurſions, are principally upon thoſe declining, conſumptive, aſthmatick, of diſeaſed lungs, worn out conſtitutions, and aged. In ſuch forlorn complaints, catarrhal influenza has haſtened the final diſſolution ſooner than it would otherwiſe have happened. In ſome, from neglect or irregularity, it has excited conſumption, or pulmonick inflammation: in others, recovering from fevers, and convaleſcents of various deſcriptions, it has occaſioned relapſes. Theſe obſervations are alſo applicable to ſimple catarrh ſkirmiſhing in leſs formidable inroads. Frequent relapſes, from imprudence, in perſons of phthiſical or aſthmatick conſtitutions, may expedite the inflammation of latent tubercles; or in aged perſons ſubject to pituitous coughs, ſpurious peripneumony.

The prediſpoſing and occaſional cauſes of catarrh are, the cutaneous perſpiration and pulmonary exhalation ſuddenly checked; cold moiſt atmoſphere; ſudden atmoſpherick changes; cold habitations and beds; wet feet; the head or breaſt expoſed or naked; thin ragged cloathing; exceſſive effeminacy and warm rooms; epidemick ſtate of the air.

Hooping Cough, chincough, tuſſis convulſiva. In the London regiſters, hooping cough and cough are confounded, and conjointly make no inconſiderable augmentation to the funerals. By the records of Dr. Armſtrong in the diſpenſary of infant poor, of 732 caſes of hooping cough, only 25 died; that is, about $3\frac{1}{2}$ *per cent.* or 1 of 33. But this, probably, is too favourable a repreſentation as a general ſcale of mortality. It is an epidemick and contagious diſeaſe, and is generally prevalent in infancy and adoleſcence, and but once in life; and is not confined to any particular ſeaſon. Its beginning reſembles a ſlight catarrh, continuing ſome days, or even weeks, before the formation and maturity of the convulſive paroxiſms. Theſe conſiſt of many ſucceſſive expiratory motions, ſucceeded by a full inſpiration and pulmonick gulp, which ruſhing through the glottis, makes a loud hooping ſound. The duration of theſe paroxiſms, is from one to ſeveral minutes, in which the child's face is turgid with blood, tears trickle down the cheeks, and it ſeems almoſt in the agony of ſuffocation. The pneumonick convulſions vary in their recurrence: they may return, frequently, in the courſe of twenty-four hours: and thus may continue to perſecute from one to ſeveral months. Throughout, the ſenſes are not injured; nor in the beginning the appetite; and in the intervals, children return to their amuſements as if nothing had happened.

The younger the child there is more danger; as alſo in thoſe born of phthiſical or aſthmatic parents, or in a ſtate of debility, when ſeized with the hooping cough. When it begins in the form of catarrh, and is attended with fever, difficulty of breathing, and little expectoration, it may prove fatal in the early immature ſtages, unleſs the convulſive cough ſupervenes, and is accompanied with copious expectoration. After ſome continuance of the diſeaſe, fever, with nocturnal exacerbation and difficult reſpiration, ſometimes occur, and always with danger: violent paroxiſms of coughing have excited epilepſy, convulſions, apoplexy, or ſuffocation; but fever, dyſpnœa, and pulmonick inflammation are to be moſt dreaded. With moderate expectoration the paroxiſms are neither frequent nor violent: but expectoration in either extremes of ſcantineſs or exceſs are both unpropitious, more eſpecially with dyſpnœa. Paroxiſms terminated by vomiting, and ſucceeded by craving for food, are favourable omens; and recovery may be predicted by longer intervals from coughing, and ſhorter paroxiſms; by reſtitu on of natural appetite and reſpiration, of tranquil ſleep, of fecal excretion, by evaneſcence of fever, and recruit of ſtrength.

The prediſpoſing and occaſional cauſes of hooping cough are, a certain epidemick ſtate of the air or ſpecifick contagion, the nature of which, and in truth of the diſeaſe beyond empirical obſervation, are as yet very imperfectly underſtood.

Croup, ſuffocatio ſtridula. This diſeaſe has been particularly diſcriminated by modern authors. It is principally inimical to children, but ſeldom until after ablactation; and never after the age of twelve, or of puberty at the utmoſt: it may attack the ſame child more than once: it is moſt frequent in winter and ſpring; and is not contagious nor general amongſt the community. It commonly invades like a catarrh; and ſometimes with its own permanent features, which are ſudden paroxiſms, as in ſpaſmodick aſthma, of laborious ſtruggling reſpiration, and wheezing; the ſenſes and appetite, during the intervals, remaining unimpaired.

It is always dangerous, infinitely more ſo than the preceding diſeaſe: ſtrangulation and death may ſuddenly enſue on the third, fourth, or fifth day, and perhaps when no ſuch event was ſuſpected. The prediſpoſing and occaſional cauſes of croup are yet the ſubject of litigation; whether inflammatory, or ſpaſmodick, or a combination of both. On diſſection, mucus accumulated and inſpiſſated has been found lining the larynx.

C H A P. VII.

A Miſcellaneous cluſter of diſeaſes are now to be developed. In the majority of theſe, however, ſome few general features of affinity may be traced: ſuch as their affecting, directly or collaterally, the head, the brain, or its numerous diverging chords, the nerves; or the inherent muſcular energy. But in many other circumſtances of cauſe, diagnoſtick, prognoſtick, and therapeutick, they are diſunited. And in every poſſible arrangement ſuch defects are irremediable.

Headach. The London regiſters neither convey an adequate repreſentation of cephallalgick fatality, and far leſs of its contentious torture of the human ſpecies. No parts of the human organization are more prone to tranſitory interruption and diſorder than the head and ſtomach: between the two there is a cloſe connubial ſympathy: to theſe two important centers many other maladies and remote perturbations converge, or reverberate their affliction. We here treat of headach as a primary diſeaſe; or at leaſt as the principal ſymptom. From this calamity, in the extreme, the lives of many are rendered wretched. Headach has been ſubdivided by authors into the idiopathick, ſymptomatick, general, local, internal, external, chronick, periodick, and temporary; into cephalea, cephalalgia, hemicrania, clavus, megrim. In the ſeat, duration, recurrence, and pain, there are many varieties and gradations.

The

The predispoſing and occaſional cauſes of headachs are, hereditary; ſanguineous or pituitous plethora, general or local; ſuppreſſion of habitual hemorrhages, as menſtrual, hemorrhoidal, naſal; checked perſpiration; cold feet; inſufficient perſpiration, and obſtructed cutaneous pores; foul, diſordered ſtomach; food or drink diſagreeing; gluttony; ebriety; unwholeſome quality of fermented or diſtilled liquors from accident or deſign; coſtiveneſs; violent exerciſe of body or mind, voice and lungs; immoderate determination of blood to the head from cauſes corporeal or mental; much ſtooping of the head; diſagreeable paſſions and anxiety of mind, exaſperating or depreſſing; ſtudy in exceſs; ſtate of the winds and weather; of the points from whence winds blow; the variations in the barometer and electrometer; the muddineſs and fogs of the atmoſphere; lunar; cold; heat; foul air; crowded rooms, theatres, and other aſſemblages of mankind for amuſement or buſineſs; offenſive ſmells and vapours; fainting; inanition; exceſſive evacuations; intermittent; rheumatick; arthritick, hyſterical; nervous; ſcorbutick; impure blood; cachexy; venereal; caries of the ſkull; diſeaſes in the diploe; abſceſs, inſects, or inflammation in the frontal, ethmoidal, or ſphenoidal ſinuſſes; firſt branch of the fifth pair of nerves particularly affected; carious teeth; various diſeaſes within the brain; external injuries; ſymptomatick in fevers, hydrocephalus, and many other diſeaſes beſides thoſe above enumerated.

Naſal Hemorrhage predominates principally in the adoleſcent age, and towards puberty, and more

more amongſt the male ſex: it is generally periodical, and from one noſtril, and either in ſlight or profuſe torrents. After puberty it commonly abates, and ſome years later ceaſes. It is ſeldom immediately fatal, and more dangerous diſeaſes have followed its raſh ſuppreſſion.

Night Mare, incubus, ephialtis, pavor nocturnus. Oppreſſed breathing during ſleep and ſenſation of load in the breaſt, and of ſuffocation; terrifick dreams, fantaſies, apparitions, viſionary encounters, and dangers; by which the perſon is at length awaked in agitation, palpitation, and ſweats. It attacks generally the dormant in a ſupine poſture.

The prediſpoſing and occaſional cauſes of night mare are, plethora; heavy ſuppers; ventricular crudity, indigeſtion, gluttony, flatulence; worms; the head laid low in bed; intenſe application of mind, and various paſſions: ſymptomatick in ſome fevers, in hyſtericks, hypochondriaſm, hydrocephalus, hydrothorax, aneuriſm, and polypi; ſometimes is a prelude of apoplexy, epilepſy, &c.

Apoplexy. Under this we ſhall aggroup ſeveral inferior ſpecies of ſtupor and vortex in the imperial ſeat of reaſon and motion; as lethargy, coma, carus, cataphora, vertigo. By apoplexy and ſuddenly, in the London regiſters, between one *eightieth* and *ninetieth* part of the community ſeem to be deſtroyed: and this mortality ſhould be magnified by the addition of many who are ſimply reported as found dead. In the laſt 30 years of the preceding century, apoplexy and ſuddenly ſtands at 3010: lethargy at 488: and megrims now omitted at 45. This thunderbolt

derbolt of death, or in the phraſe of one of the Britiſh poets, "that knocketh man down as "butcher felleth ox," is principally hoſtile to thoſe advanced in years, and the aged: to thoſe more eſpecially of large heads and ſhort necks, of corpulent habits, and indolent life; to the full feeders, or the addicted to frequent intoxication. Medical obſervations alſo repreſent it as affecting more of the male than the female ſex; as more predominant in winter and ſpring, eſpecially on vernal heat ſucceeding winter cold; or moiſt rainy weather ſupplanting cold, and *vice verſa*. It is alſo ſaid to be more general and fatal in the city than the country. Some information in this diſeaſe might be gleaned from diſpenſaries, none, it is obvious, from hoſpitals; but moſt of all from the ſcattered obſervations of individuals, were they collected together.

Apoplexy may attack ſuddenly; in other caſes it is preceded days, weeks, or even months, before the ſhock, by ſome injury or diſorder of either the external or internal ſenſes, or of ſome of the numerous muſcular functions, or of the countenance, voice, or ſpeech. In the paroxiſm, the patient, inſtantaneouſly ſtunned, falls down, with ſuſpenſion of the functions of the external and internal ſenſes, of voluntary motion, and of voice and ſpeech; and with muſcular relaxation; at the ſame time the pulſe and reſpiration remain nearly in the natural ſtate, excepting that there is generally a ſtertor in breathing, reſembling a profound ſleep from groſs intoxication; and alſo, as in moſt ſoporous diſeaſes, the circulation ſlow. Theſe unmoleſted

molested functions of the heart and lungs distinguish it from syncope. In the duration and severity of the symptoms, there are different gradations.

It often proves fatal at the first stroke: few can survive many attacks. Death, recovery, or transition into palsy, are generally decided within seven days. The less the functions of internal and external sense, and of voluntary motions are injured, our hopes are more flattering. In magnitude of danger, perhaps no other disease can contend with this formidable antagonist: but I shall leave it to others to graduate the apoplectick scale. Some recover; in others it ends in death or hemiplegy, which is but a sad alternative and capitulation for life: and too frequently is accompanied with some lesion of the mental functions. Even of those who recover, they are in danger of relapses from intemperance, and errors in the non-naturals.

Of Lethargy, Coma, Carus, Cataphora. These denote different degrees of profound deep sleep without delirium. Authors have often confounded them with the febrile class, especially the "*lusus naturæ*" of remittents. To this irresistible torpor and drowsiness, even at meals or in conversation, many corpulent and fat persons are subject. The vertigo is commonly fugacious, and momentary; and in some diseases is symptomatick: sometimes it is periodical and chronic. The prognosticks of all may be deduced from that of apoplexy.

Of the predisposing and occasional causes of apoplexy, lethargy, coma, carus, cataphora, and vertigo: these are hereditary; short neck; plethora,

plethora, general or partial, ſanguine or ſerous, eſpecially ſanguineous plethora in the veſſels of the brain; tight neckcloaths; preſſure on the deſcending aorta, cava; ſerous or ſanguineous exudations or extravaſations in the brain; compreſſion of the medullary ſubſtance, or of the origin of the nerves; ſuppreſſion of habitual evacuations or hemorrhages, naſal or hemorrhoidal; habitual veneſection neglected; old ulcers dried up; full and long continued inſpiration loading the veſſels of the head; blood forced on the brain by violent efforts of coughing, vomiting, fecal expulſion, exerciſe, venery, ſtooping the head; ſalivation ſuddenly ſuppreſſed by cold; foul ſtomach, gluttony, ſurfeits, luxurious living, and ſedentary life; fatneſs, corpulency; intoxication, ſottiſh potations; violent paſſions of mind iraſcible or ſtimulating, and alſo depreſſing, as anger, ambition, chronic melancholy and cares; intenſe meditation and ſtudy; intemperate luſt in old age; noxious vapour from liquors in fermentation, from charcoal, quicklime, and new-plaſtered walls; particular effluvia and odours concentrated in large quantity; crowded rooms filled with animal ſteams from the lungs; thunder; ſometimes epidemick ſtate of the air and elements, or perhaps celeſtial influences not yet explained; intenſe cold; warm baths; rarefaction and expanſion of the blood; inſolation; ſome narcotick poiſons, as opium, hyoſcyamus, cicuta, laurus, belladonna, and ſome fungi: obſtructed circulation through the lungs and heart, from aſthma, polypi, oſſifications of the large blood veſſels or valves, and particularly of the right ventricle; external in-

juries

juries of the head; concuſſion, fractures. The moſt frequent cauſe is, accumulation and congeſtion of blood in the brain: but ſometimes, on diſſection, no diſeaſe is diſcernible; and effuſions in the brain do not always inflict apoplexy.

Of vertigo, the cauſes are ſeveral of thoſe juſt enumerated: the principal plethora, ſuppreſſed hemorrhages; ſuppreſſed perſpiration; luxurious diet, gluttony, ſomnolency; foul or diſordered ſtomach; coſtiveneſs; intoxication; narcotick and tobacco fumes; unremitting attention of mind to ſtudy or buſineſs; reſtleſſneſs, mental diſtreſs; hunger, inanition, debility; obſtructions and diſeaſes in the retina or optick nerves.

Palſy. Paralyſis, hemiplegia, paraplegia. During the laſt thirty years of the preceding century, paralytick mortality is only 630 in the London bills; but in the preſent century is doubled and trebled; and ſome part of this ſurge can be readily accounted for by the multiplication of the mechanical arts, in which lead and quickſilver are employed. At preſent, its mortality ſeems to ſtand in the proportion of one third or fourth to that of apoplexy. Of 310 patients afflicted with palſy and hemiplegy, and admitted in the courſe of 10 years into the Bath hoſpital, 57 were cured; that is, 18 *per cent.* or 1 of $5\frac{1}{2}$; there died 15, or 5 *per cent.*; and the remainder were found incurable and diſcharged, or received ſome trifling relief; and ſeveral of theſe might be added to the dead liſt. I doubt whether by the remedies of the ſhops we are ſo ſucceſsful againſt this crippling foe: by by which a conſiderable number of the community are rendered helpleſs and decrepit; but the adult and aged infinitely more than the young and adoleſcent.

Palſy and apoplexy often alternate: ſevere apoplectick ſtrokes, if not immediately fatal, frequently remit, and paſs into palſy: or the cataſtrophe may originate in hemiplegy, which is the moſt frequent form of palſy; and when fatal, it is through the apoplectick exploſion. In palſy there is more or leſs diminution or privation of muſcular motion and feeling, without pain or fever, or injury of appetite. This may affect the muſcles of voluntary and of involuntary motion; the whole, or only a portion of each: as muſcular impotency of one ſide, or half of the body; of one or both of the lower or upper extremities; or of ſome ſmaller muſcular portion of the face, eyelids, tongue, œſophagus, ſtomach, inteſtines, ſphincters of the bladder and anus, penis, bladder, kidneys, heart. Under this deplorable calamity many linger years; ſome confined like a ſhellfiſh, and motionleſs; others crawling upon crutches. Tremor may be ranked as an inferior vaſſal of palſy. The *Berbiers* of Indoſtan have alſo ſome affinity. The bedridden are alſo paralytic cripples.

The prediſpoſing and occaſional cauſes of palſy are moſt of thoſe of apoplexy; various diſeaſes of the cerebrum, cerebellum, and medulla oblongata; diſeaſes of the inherent muſcular power; vapours from lead, mercury, arſenick; colica ſaturnina; compreſſion of nerves; abſceſſes in the lumbar vertebræ; falls, external injuries, blows on the head or loins, luxations

or

or ſprains of the lumbar vertebræ; ſpinal dropſy; fractures; venery. Of tremor many of the cauſes of apoplexy and palſy; hereditary; old age and decay of the inherent nervous and muſcular energy; compreſſion or obſtruction of the nerves; poiſons; opium; employments in lead and mercury; ebriety; ſuppreſſed evacuations; ſanguine plethora; repelled cutaneous eruptions; lurking gout; general debility; external injuries; warm fluids; ſtrong tea; exceſs of venery; long watching; anxiety; paſſions of mind; ſedentary life; exceſſive evacuations.

Epilepſy. Morbus ſacer, demoniacus, caducus, falling-ſickneſs. In the laſt thirty years of the preceding century, 35 deaths only are marked in the London bills to epilepſy; and in the firſt forty-five years of the preſent century, they dwindle to 13: at preſent the title and diſeaſe is omitted. Medical men know, that no inconſiderable number of the community are tormented with this frightful convulſion, which the ancient Jews could only aſcribe to the malicious rancour of an infernal devil. In this inſtance alſo, profeſſional experience and erudition muſt interfere and correct the omiſſions of the publick regiſters. We are certain, that epilepſy is much more deſtructive to the ſprings of life: perhaps it is caſt by the reporters into either the apoplectick or convulſive abyſs. It is alledged to be more frequent amongſt the male than female ſex; and in infancy, in thoſe of delicate conſtitutions, lax habit, acute, nervous and muſcular irritability. *Vid.* Convulſions.

By the epileptick whirlwind the patient is ſuddenly thrown upon the ground, and agitated with univerſal convulſions. In moſt, the aſpect then is horrible, nor does any other diſeaſe exhibit more truculent ſpectacles. After ſome few minutes, very rarely hours, a pacification enſues, and abdication of the epileptick demon; and the patient liberated, riſes up of his own accord, languid and dejected; and nearly in the exerciſe of all his uſual faculties; which is not the caſe in apoplexy. In the ſeverity and duration, but ſtill more in the repetition of the paroxiſms, there is prodigious variation: in ſome they are erratick and irregular; in others, they are periodical, and at various intervals; in diurnal paroxiſms, ſynchronous with the tides; monthly with the lunar revolutions; equinoctial; annual. It is often a chronic diſeaſe, and then much leſs inimical to life than might be expected from ſuch a univerſal commotion. But in infancy, epilepſy and convulſions are the moſt atrocious of the morbid murderers. Sometimes it ceaſes after puberty. In old perſons, or where there is no previous warning of the approaching paroxiſms, the proſpects are deplorable: reiterated epileptick ſhocks often make breaches in the internal receſſes of the ſenſes; hence inſanity, apoplexy, palſy, idiotiſm. This convulſion is ſometimes feigned by begging impoſtors.

The prediſpoſing and occaſional cauſes of epilepſy are, hereditary, peculiar original organization, eſpecially of the brain and its appendages: plethora, fright, terror, horror, anxiety and paſſions of mind, exceſs of venery, ſtudy: in infancy from paſſionate drunken nurſes, foul ſtomach, acidity, acrid bile, worms, dentition; from

from raſh repulſion or drying up of ſcald head, or ulcers; external injuries of the head; various diſeaſes within the brain, or in the nervous chords; ebriety; difficult parturition; hyſtericks; cachexy, dregs of intermittent fevers; irritability and ſenſibility in morbid extreme; nervous ſympathy and motory vibrations; force of habit; offenſive odours; poiſons, narcoticks. In thoſe of epileptick temperament and prediſpoſition, paroxiſms are liable to be recalled by heat, ventricular crudity, intoxication, anxiety and paſſions of mind, terror, proſpect of precipices, &c.

Tetanus, emproſthotonus, opiſthotonus, locked jaw, triſmus. This is not a frequent diſeaſe in Britain, nor in Europe: it is far more univerſal and fatal in the tropical regions, and in the warmeſt ſeaſons of thoſe zones. In ſuch climates tetanus, and all the train of ſpaſmodick and convulſive diſeaſes rage with more inveterate rancour and devaſtation: there the ſlighteſt wound or ſcratch will frequently occaſion a locked jaw; and this ſometimes happens after the wound is healed. It afflicts more adults than youth; and, as is reported, more males than females. The emproſthotonus, or head bent forward on the breaſt, is much leſs frequent than the reverſe. It may prove fatal in a few hours; generally, if not relieved, in a few days; and rarely is protracted beyond fourteen. Its danger is increaſed from the ſudden impetuoſity of the aſſault, and from wounded nerves: the final tragedy is cloſed by convulſions. Until of late years, and the diſcovery of more effectual remedies, few recovered. Authors alſo deſcribe a ſpaſm of the lower jaw, and difficulty of ſuction, to which infants are ſubject, and which they term tetanus and triſmus.

The prediſpoſing and occaſional cauſes of tetanus and its ſpecies, are wounds, particularly of the fingers and toes; ſurgical operations, fractures, luxations, burns, injuries of a nervous, tendinous and ſenſible part, bruiſed teſticle; ſuppuration, abſceſs; cold and moiſture applied to the body when heated; ſudden ſuppreſſion of perſpiration; ſudden viciſſitudes of heat and cold; repletion, foul ſtomach and inteſtines in infants; dentition; bile in the ſtomach; worms; poiſons; ebriety; exceſſive evacuations, hemorrhages; ſuppreſſed ſalutary evacuations, exanthemata and cutaneous eruptions; abortion; difficult parturition; violent mental emotion; angina; lurking gout; hemorrhoides; hypochondriaſm, hyſtericks, melancholy. In many of theſe it is merely ſymptomatick.

Spaſms and cramps are idiopathick as well as ſymptomatick; fugacious, or more fixed and conſtant; with different gradations of pain and torture; and may affect various portions of the external and of the internal muſcular fibres, of the head, neck, face, eye, lower jaw, lips, arms, hands, fingers, thighs, legs, feet, penis, tongue, fauces, pharynx, œſophagus, lungs, ſtomach, inteſtines, kidneys, ureters, bladder.

St. Vitus's Dance. Chorea ſancti Viti. This very uncommon diſeaſe, a compound of ſpaſm and palſy, or rather hemiplegy, and accompanied with extraordinary convulſive geſticulations of the affected arm, may afflict either of the ſexes about the period of adoleſcence and

2 puberty;

puberty; rarely afterwards. The paroxiſms vary in duration and frequency: ſometimes they are terminated in half an hour: ſometimes they continue ſeveral days, rarely a week, without intermiſſion: ſometimes they recur ſeveral times daily, leaving behind debility and weakneſs. The prediſpoſing and occaſional cauſes are moſtly unknown: ſometimes worms.

Catalepſis, and extaſis. It falls to the lot of very few phyſicians, to ſee a ſingle inſtance of this phenomenon, a living ſtatue fixed in whatever ſituation and poſture they happen to be in when ſeized; with the legs and arms flexible. The duration of the paroxiſm is from a minute to hours, very rarely days. In the Extaſis ſtrange viſions are ſeen: and of theſe trances there are extraordinary inſtances on record. It may be complicated with ſomnambuliſmus, and hyſtericks. The cauſes of both are deep meditation, fanaticiſm, mental paſſions, intenſe cold, worms, foul ſtomach, ſuppreſſed evacuations: extacy has been feigned by impoſtors.

Fainting and aſphyxy: ſyncope, leipothymia, aſphyxia; idiopathick, ſymptomatick. In ſyncope the action of the heart and of reſpiration become conſiderably weaker than uſual, or for a ſhort time ſuſpended: the pulſe and breathing are ſometimes ſo weak as to be imperceptible; the countenance is pale and cold. In the gradation and duration of vital ſuſpenſion, there are diverſities: but after the lapſe of a few or more minutes they gradually revive. This partial ceſſation of the vital functions diſtinguiſhes it, at the firſt glance, from apoplexy. Aſphyxy is only a more violent degree of ſyncope in which the entire human machinery is ſtopped: the counterfeit of death; but in which there are embers capable of being fanned and vivified into vital renovation. Vid. Hyſtericks.

The prediſpoſing and occaſional cauſes of ſyncope and aſphyxy, idiopathiek and ſymptomatick are, profuſe evacuations and hemorrhages; veneſection; tapping the abdomen in aſcites; ſtrong emeticks and purgatives; exhauſted ſtrength; violent exertions of ſtrength, or muſcular action; exceſſive fatigue; venery in exceſs; ſudden terror or joy, or other mental emotions; intenſe anxiety; ſevere pain; offenſive ſmells; foul air; cloſe rooms and crowds, and the air contaminated with their breath and effluvia; charcoal fumes; foul ſtagnant confined air, and gas of old damp pits, wells, ſubterranean caverns, mines; mephitick vapours from fermenting liquors in conſiderable quantity; lightening, thunder-ſhocks; exceſſive heat; exceſſive cold; ſanguineous plethora; various diſeaſes of the ſtomach; poiſons, narcoticks; repelled cutaneous eruptions; hyſterick, ſcorbutick, arthritick, febrile; wounds or blows on the head, ſpine, or ſtomach: ſevere labour and parturition, in which the infant's head and brain is compreſſed, injured, or mouldſhot, or the navel-ſtring compreſſed, and the circulation interrupted; hydrocephalus: internal aneuriſm, polypi of the heart, or large arterial trunks; rupture of large blood veſſels, or of internal abſceſs; palſy of the heart, dropſy of the pericardium; gangrene; drowning; hanging.

Palpitation of the Heart. Chronic is here meant, not tranſitory, which may occur on every

ſudden

ſudden emotion of body or mind. In this the contraction of the heart is with outrageous rapidity and force, and often with audible ſtrokes againſt the ribs, and with intermittent pulſe. It is generally periodical; and by continuance, it is evident that, from the convulſion of this important organ, the entire ſubordinate ſeries of hydraulick offices, together with thoſe of ſenſe and motion, muſt ſhare in the diſorder.

The prediſpoſing and occaſional cauſes are, plethora; repletion, intemperance in food or drink; ſuppreſſion of habitual evacuations; exceſſive evacuations; inanition; paſſions of mind, long continued grief, terror, venery, pain, anxiety; thirſt, immoderate exerciſe, light cloathing; extreme irritability, peculiar irritability of the heart, and debility, ſpaſm; preſſure on the arota; aneuriſm; oſſification and ſtraitneſs of the aorta; tumors about the great veſſels; polypi; dropſy of the pericardium; impeded reſpiration and circulation through the lungs; broken ribs; weak diſordered ſtomach, flatulence; diſeaſes of the abdominal viſcera; ſweat of the feet, ulcers, ſcabs prematurely repreſſed; cachexy; hyſterick, hypochondriack, melancholick, ſcorbutick, arthritick, atrabilarious, inflammatory. Vid. Hyſtericks.

Polypi of the Heart, internal Aneuriſm, and Oſſification. Polypi of the heart are ſolid coagulums of blood, of a firm or fleſhy conſiſtence: aneuriſm a diſtention and weakneſs, and partial enlargement or bulge in ſome portion of the arterial coats. The uſual ſeat of the firſt is in the auricles and ventricles; of the ſecond, in the large trunks, and more about their origin. Oſſification of the valves, and of the aorta, or the ſmaller branches, is more frequent in old age. The ſymptoms of polypi and aneuriſm are often ambiguous; moſt of them are common to ſome other pneumonick diſeaſes. Theſe, together with ſyncope and aſphxy, no doubt, make a part of the ſudden deaths, and ſome other caſualties in the London regiſters.

Hypochondriaſm, hips, ſpleen, and vapours, imaginary maladies. This chronic valetudinary infatuation is very frequent in our iſland: it occurs principally in the adult and middle age; in the male more than in the female ſex, eſpecially in thoſe of melancholick temperaments; and much more amongſt perſons of independent fortunes, and of literary and ſedentary profeſſions, than the exerciſed and induſtrious. Vapours are often complicated with diſeaſes of the ſtomach, hyſtericks, melancholy. But in the true hypochondriaſm, the valetudinary dyſpepſy, and diſeaſes of the digeſtive organs, ſeem rather a natural conſequence and ſequel of ſuch temperament: beſides, in dyſpepſy the mental perturbation is ſlight; it is alſo a far more univerſal diſeaſe than hypochondriaſm, affecting equally both ſexes; and the young as well as the old; and has fewer of the miſanthropic features.

Hypochondriacks feel, or imagine they feel, all diſeaſes; againſt theſe they combat with a thouſand remedies, and exhauſt the whole pharmaceutical rotine. They exaggerate with minute narrative theſe morbid phantoms, which no other perſon can perceive, nor account for; examining their pulſe, fatiguing and harraſſing their phyſicians, viſitors, and domeſticks; on the ſlighteſt grounds haunted with apprehenſive forebodings

forebodings of misfortunes, misery, and death; and in the utmost anxiety about the event, at the time perhaps that the appetite is not much impaired: in most things, however, their judgment is correct; their health and diseases excepted, which are the constant objects of their fears, and despondency.

By such anxious solicitude, and passive submission to fanciful and imperative chimeras, a luxuriant brood of symptoms, like irregular hystericks, are engendered: they at length convert, or at least aggravate, accelerate, and multiply imaginary into real evils, deranging the complicated offices of digestion, of circulation, of excretion and secretion, and of the mental functions. It sometimes ceases, or at least abates weeks and months, recurring in periodical exacerbations on any exciting cause or mental distress, intemperance, or vicissitudes and irregularity of the seasons. It is not immediately dangerous to life; but when of inveterate continuance, may terminate in insanity, cachexy, jaundice, dropsy, tympany, consumption.

The predisposing and occasional causes of hypochondriasm are morbid extreme of sensibility; hereditary; various depressing passions of mind; studious sedentary life and abstruse meditation; retirement to an inactive after a bustling busy life; excess of venery, manustupration; wealth, indolence, transient, unsatisfactory amusements; revels in pleasures, and dissipation to satiety; intemperance in food or drink, gross diet and drink; suppression of usual and salutary evacuations, as menses, hemorrhoids; repulsion of cutaneous eruptions; obstruction in the circulation

lation through the vena porta and liver, and in the biliary ſecretion; obſtruction in the abdominal viſcera; debility in the ſtomach and inteſtines, and conſequently vitiated chyle; pituita in exceſs; worms; irregular gout; hyſtericks; intermittent fever; ſcurvy; November fogs, eaſterly winds, ſirocco winds; foggy atmoſphere.

Inſanity, lunacy, mania, melancholia, and complex inſanity. During the preceding century, diſtracted and lunatick was the term in the London regiſters; and in the laſt thirty years of that century, amounted in the funerals to 544; but in the preſent century, are quadruple. We muſt reflect, that two of the largeſt lunatick hoſpitals in Europe are erected in this metropolis, excluſive of ſeveral private madhouſes; all of which are of late years enlarged and multiplied in London and its ſuburbs. Into theſe publick and private receptacles many lunaticks, from ſundry parts of the kingdom, are congregated; amounting in all, to upwards of one thouſand. Perhaps thoſe whom nature originally, or diſeaſe branded as idiots, are alſo included in the lunatick catalogue of mortality. The coroner's inqueſt generally returns ſuicides as lunaticks, after reciting the mode of their death; but the ſearcher's reports in the bills of mortality, have invariably ranged lunatick and ſelf-murder under two diſtinct heads. I have reaſon to believe that many lunatick deaths in London are not reported, from their being interred in diſſenting and unregiſtered burying grounds, or in other places of interment without the verge of the bills; from others intentionally ſuppreſſed, and a conſiderable remnant,

perhaps

perhaps as many more, ſunk amongſt the ſuicides and drowned. It is probable, that in lunaticks and ſuicides, our nation may challenge any other in Europe, whether in modern or in ancient times.

In illuſtrating this diſeaſe, above all others ſo little underſtood by the medical profeſſion, or, in truth, by the greateſt part of the authors on the ſubject, I ſhall rather treſpaſs beyond the limits of a ſyſtematick ſurvey. I was anxious to extend my inquiries to a vaſt variety of particulars, not one of which could be learned from the crowd of authors, good, bad, and indifferent, whom I peruſed for this purpoſe, from the remote era of the Greek and Roman Catholicon, the Hellebore, down to the preſent time. From Bedlam, the largeſt palace and congregation of inſane in any part of the globe; and from its valuable, but hitherto dormant archives, I ſhall attempt to eſtabliſh all the leading and important data, by analyzing its internal hiſtory and tranſactions during fifteen years, or half a generation; which is ſufficient to decide every ambiguity nearly as well as half a century. The materials are extracted from many volumes; and are condenſed, claſſed, and arranged into conciſe tables, with no little trouble and fatigue to the author.

For theſe regiſters I am indebted to the venerable and learned phyſician of Bedlam, Dr. Monro, and to his ſon; and more eſpecially to Mr. Gozna, the apothecary of Bedlam, whoſe learning and curioſity induced him to keep a *private* regiſter of all the patients; with all which Mr. Gozna moſt obligingly furniſhed

me;

me; and upon which, as incontrovertible data, I have founded and collected all the following tables and propositions. Since the first edition of this book, I have again and again examined, compared, and digested the registers, with very laborious and perplexing scrutiny. I may with safety assert, that mine are the only numerical and certain data that ever have been published in any age or country, by which to calculate the probabilities of recovery, of death, and of relapse in every species and stage of insanity, and in every age.

Nine different TABLES, demonstrating, first, the total number of insane, and the proportion of male and female patients that were admitted into Bedlam, during fifteen years, from 1772 to 1787: secondly, the intervals of time elapsed from the first unequivocal manifestation of the mental derangement, until their admission into Bedlam, divided into three periods, from one week to the end of six months, from six to the end of twelve months, and from one year upwards: thirdly, the comparative proportion of insane throughout the different intervals or stages of life: fourthly, the comparative proportion of the not mischievous, of the mischievous, together with those who attempted suicide, and also of the few who committed murders: fifthly, the comparative proportion, including all ages of cured, incurable, and dead: sixthly, the principal, occasional, and remote causes of insanity; together with the comparative proportion of cured, incurable, and dead, as influenced by each of those different causes: seventhly, the

the comparative proportion of cured, incurable, and dead, as influenced by youth and by age: eighthly, the comparative proportion of cured and incurable after 1, 2, 3, or 4 years and upwards, from the first manifestation and uninterrupted perseverance of the malady, and demonstrating the prospects of cure, as influenced by the different duration of insanity: ninthly, the periods of life when hereditary insanity usually first breaks out.

TABLE I.

A short Table, demonstrating the proportion of insane patients admitted into Bedlam from 1772 to 1787: the males and females are nearly equal in number.

Total number insane 2829.

TABLE II.

The intervals of time elapsed from the first unequivocal manifestation of the mental derangement, until their admission into Bedlam, divided into three intervals, from one week to the end of six months; from the end of six to twelve months; from one year to ten, or more.

	Time elapsed before admission.		Numb. admitted.
Insane admitted	under 7 months	—	1926
	From the end of 6 to 12 months		324
	After 1 year and upwards	—	579
	Total	—	2829

TABLE

TABLE III.

The comparative proportion of inſane admitted into Bedlam, diſtinguiſhed into the not miſchievous, the miſchievous, together with thoſe who attempted ſuicide, and alſo the few who committed murders.

Inſane not miſchievous	——	1320
Miſchievous	——	1097
Attempted ſuicide	——	402
Committed murders	——	20
Total	——	2819

TABLE IV.

The comparative proportion of inſane throughout the different intervals or ſtages of life, and founded on the Bedlam regiſters.

Years of age.		Numb. inſane.
Inſane under 10 years	——	1
From 10 to 20	——	132
20 to 30	——	813
30 to 40	——	908
40 to 50	——	632
50 to 60	——	266
60 and upwards	—	77
Total	——	2829

TABLE V.

The comparative proportion, including all ages in the groſs, of cured, incurable, and dead; founded on the Bedlam regiſters.

Inſane cured	——	925
Incurable	——	1674
Dead	——	230
Total	——	2829

TABLE

TABLE VI.

The principal, occafional, and remote caufes of infanity, together with the comparative proportion of cured, incurable, and dead, as influenced by each of thefe different caufes; and alfo the proportion of relapfes: founded on the Bedlam regifters.

The principal occafional, and remote caufes of infanity; and proportion of relapfes.	Total number of infane from each of the different caufes.	Cured	Incurable.	Dead.
Misfortunes, troubles, difappointments, grief, vexation, loffes, croffes, jealoufy, ill-ufage, anxiety, defpair, diftrefs	383	109	235	39
Religion and methodifm —	166	54	90	22
Frights — —	96	38	51	7
Love — —	136	50	80	6
Study — —	40	10	27	3
Pride — —	23	2	20	1
Drink — —	111	31	68	12
Parturition — —	145	66	69	10
Fever — —	212	100	86	26
Family and hereditary —	213	90	103	20
Venereal — —	24	10	11	3
Contufion, fracture, and fall	13	8	5	0
Obftruction — —	18	8	5	
Ulcer and fcab dried up —	7			
Relapfes from all the preceding caufes, and alfo from preceding lefion by infanity —	1205	508	623	74
Total —	2829			

TABLE

TABLE VII.

The comparative proportion of cured, incurable, and dead, as influenced by youth and by age; and founded on the Bedlam regiſters.

Comparative ages.	Total number inſane at theſe ages.	Cured.	Incurable.	Dead.
The inſane from 10 to 20 years of age —	132	74	54	4
The inſane from 30 to 40 years of age —	908	276	550	82
The inſane from 50 to 60 years of age —	266	62	174	30

TABLE VIII.

The comparative proportion of inſane cured after 1, 2, 3, 4, or more years manifeſtation, and uninterrupted perſeverance of the malady; and demonſtrating the proſpects of cure, as influenced by the different duration of inſanity: founded on the Bedlam regiſters.

Total inſane 1, 2, 3, 4, 5, 6 years and upwards.	Time elapſed before admiſſion.	Numbers cured.
Of the above admitted 256	From 1 to 2 years —	33
323	From 2 to 3 years —	6
	3 to 4 years —	2
	4 to 5 years —	1
	After 5 and upwards	000
Total — 579		

TABLE

TABLE IX.

The periods of life when hereditary inſanity uſually firſt breaks out: founded on the Bedlam regiſters.

Comparative ages.		Numb. inſane.
From 10 to 20 years of age	—	12
20 to 30	———	74
30 to 40	———	64
40 to 50	———	49
50 to 60	———	9
60 to 70	———	2

Upon each of theſe Tables I ſhall now proceed, in the order of their arrangement, to found a multitude of original and uſeful propoſitions. Each ſex ſeems equally obnoxious to inſanity: at leaſt the difference is very inconſiderable, and if any, the females rather preponderate. Mr. Gozna had diſcriminated the married and ſingle; but in our general ſurvey, theſe, and ſeveral other minutiæ muſt be excluded. The uſual number, on a general average, of patients in Bedlam is 250; of which 110 are ſtationary incurables, or ſo called, male and female, who remain there until they either die, or are diſcharged for reaſons hereafter to be explained. The remainder are a moving body, upwards of 200 of whom are annually admitted, and the ſame number annually diſcharged, at various intervals of time. Thoſe whoſe caſes continue rebellious are permitted to remain one year; after which, they are either diſcharged as

 incurable,

incurable, or admitted into the hoſpital liſt of that denomination.

The ſecond Table contains information indiſpenſible, on numerous accounts, the different intervals of time elapſed from the firſt unequivocal manifeſtation of inſanity, until their admiſſion into Bedlam. This muſt be aſcertained as one of the preliminaries to the other prognoſticks reſpecting the hopes of cure, and the proportion of incurable. Of the patients ranked in the curable liſt of the hoſpital, that is not one year inſane before admiſſion, are found conſiderably more than 2 to 1 not 7 months in that predicament when received into Bedlam, and diſperſed, promiſcuouſly, in all the intervals, from 1 week to the end of 6 months. Thoſe admitted after one year's derangement of reaſon amount to nearly 1-5th of all the patients; and are uſually refuſed admiſſion, except on the incurable liſt, although a conſiderable number of ſuch caſes are not deſperate, as will hereafter appear.

The third Table exhibits the comparative proportion of the not-miſchievous, of the miſchievous, of thoſe who attempted ſuicide, and a few who committed murders. Theſe data are of the utmoſt importance in enabling us to found probable prognoſticks, and to direct the regimen and cure. Under this head alſo the general features of inſanity may be delineated. Inſanity is termed a delirium, generally without fever, at leaſt after continuing ſome time; of which mental anarchy there are innumerable ſymptoms, gradations, ſhades, ſpecies, and varieties; the enumeration of which would be as infinite

infinite as the diverſity of their faces and ideas. It has been deſcribed by authors in the two extremes of mania and melancholia; but it is ofteneſt of a complex nature, with alternating exacerbations of frenzy, and of temporary remiſſion or calm, or of melancholy; in which the violence, duration, repetition, and intervals are immenſely various. Sometimes inſanity burſts out, unexpectedly, like a ſquall of wind or thunder ſtorm; but frequently the paroxiſm is preceded days, weeks, or even months, by ſomething unuſual and different in the conduct, geſtures, looks, countenance, voice, ſpeech, paſſions, ſpirits, ſleep, appetite.

On the firſt eruption of frantick mania, the looks, voice, and geſtures are wild and impetuous; in many audacious and ferocious: they are iraſcible, impatient, and violent on any contradiction or reſtraint; and their ſtrength is prodigiouſly increaſed: they ramble with wonderful rapidity of ideas, and garrulity from one object to another, ſhouting, ſinging, laughing, ſwearing: ſome roam in incoherent rhapſody through all the regions of enchantment and romance: we obſerve maniacks in idea perſonating every object celeſtial and terreſtrial, animate and inanimate. But by ſuch numbers either attempting or committing miſchief againſt others or themſelves, it is evident, that the diſagreeable, turbulent, diſcordant, deſponding, and malevolent paſſions do very often predominate: ſome maniacks are diſtracted with malevolence, antipathy, animoſity, rancour, and revenge. In the fixed melancholia, the mind is generally rivetted upon one object and train of thought,

 about

about which they inceſſantly rave, mutter, or ponder, or emit lamentations: many are cogitative, taciturn, moroſe, or fixed like ſtatues. Some plunged into deſpair, are haunted with all the horrors of Tartarus; or even chained, in imagination, within the gloomy dungeons and inexorable bars of Cerberus.

In general, inſane perſons endure hunger, cold, nakedneſs, and want of ſleep, with aſtoniſhing perſeverance and impunity. Some obſtinately refuſe all food, and are drenched by compulſion, as horſes taking phyſick; which at length renders them more docile. Some, if indulged, are ravenous and inſatiable as wolves. During the exacerbation moſt are reſtleſs, and moſt are coſtive. Many perſons, univerſally conſidered as inſane, will however, at times, act, ſpeak, converſe, and reaſon acutely on various ſubjects, until ſome particular mental ſtring or chord is touched, or until agitated by ſome ſtrong emotions of mind, or until ſome periodical and inexplicable exacerbation of the malady. In truth, inſanity is not confined within the porticoes of Bedlam and madhouſes: we might find it ſprinkled over the earth, not only amongſt the fanaticks of Aſia, and the cloiſtered devotees of Europe, but through every rank and ſtation of civilized communities. In the definition of the diſeaſe, we may not only apply the term of chronic delirium, but of waking dreams.

Of the patients in Bedlam denominated not miſchievous, and alſo of the miſchievous, together with thoſe who attempted ſuicide, I find nearly an equal diſtribution of males and females:

males: and from all the variety of caufes, depreffing and ftimulating, I perceive mifchievous or harmlefs promifcuoufly. The mifchievous acts were of various kinds, either againft other perfons or themfelves, without difcrimination of friends, relations, or ftrangers, but with particular vindictivenefs towards their keepers, by attempting to ftab, fhoot, or injure them; by fetting fire to houfes, jumping out of windows, or into water, tearing off their clothes, obftinately rejecting fuftenance, by hanging, and a variety of ftratagems, endeavouring to deftroy their own lives. Some were mifchievous by overt acts of violence; others by threats only. Some not mifchievous at firft, have afterwards become fo, and "*vice verfa*;" and fome reported as not mifchievous, have afterwards hanged themfelves. The mifchievous actions were moft frequent at the commencement of infanity. Except during temporary exacerbations of frenzy or melancholy, the majority of patients in Bedlam walk peaceably and promifcuoufly about the wards and galleries, only that the fexes do not intermix: feparate confinement in their cells, ftrait waiftcoats, or in the ferocious maniac, handcuffs and chains, foon render them tractable and obedient. A very fmall number are kept as wild beafts, conftantly in fetters. Some, who were extremely vicious and dangerous, by time and long confinement, become harmlefs, fatuitous, and are difcharged. The attempts at fuicide are more prevalent, either amongft the permanent melancholick; or in others, during the periodical paroxifm of defpondency.

Of the miſchievous, vicious, and dangerous to others, or to themſelves, and conſtituting nearly one half of all the inſane, their recovery ſeems not in the leaſt degree retarded by that ſymptom, not excepting the attempts at ſuicide, which are nearly 1-7th of the whole inſane; nor do more of this deſcription die. Amongſt the inſane liſt of murderers there are parricides and butchers of their own offspring; the majority of whom were males, and ſome of them occur amongſt the recoveries.

The fourth Table illuſtrates the comparative proportion of inſane throughout the different ſtages or intervals of life; the comments upon which are obvious. In the ſecond period, between 10 and 20 years of age, the greateſt part of this ſmall group occurred between 15 and 20. Before puberty, therefore, there are few inſtances of inſanity. From 20 to 50 years of age, the inſane are more numerous in the proportion nearly of 7 to 1, than throughout all the other antecedent and poſterior ſtages of life united.

The fifth Table exhibits the comparative proportion in the groſs of the cured, incurable, and dead, at all ages. This is truth, but not the whole truth; and without attending to the comments a ſuperficial reader muſt be bewildered, and led to form erroneous concluſions. An ambiguous term *diſcharged* is uſed by the hoſpital; amongſt whom I found a conſiderable number reported as ſick and weak, as afflicted with epileptick fits, or with paralytick ſtrokes, and ſome with a complication of both the latter maladies, together with a ſmall number of pregnant females; the whole united amounting to

ſome

ſome hundreds, and none of them liberated from inſanity when diſcharged. All theſe I threw into the incurable liſt, as I could diſcover very few of them ever to return back again: and it is obſerved, that very few are cured without the fits alſo; and with what difficulty thoſe are removed has already appeared. Many of the diſcharged as ſick and weak, might, with equal propriety, have been added to the dead liſt, being then on the confines of the grave. We ſhould likewiſe remember, that the incurables include not only the crowd annually diſcharged from Bedlam in that forlorn ſtate, after one year's trial of the effects of medicine, but likewiſe thoſe originally entered on the incurable liſt of the hoſpital, as being more than one year inſane, and of whom the greateſt part are afterwards diſcharged amongſt the incurables.

It would appear from this Table, including the aggregate maſs of patients, that the incurable are not altogether double to the cured; and that the dead are as 1 of 13 or 14. But on theſe ſeparate heads of incurable and dead, many conſiderations and reflections preſent, tending to ſubtract from the ſuperiority of incurables to that of cured, and to reduce them nearer to an equality. Several of theſe conſiderations muſt be reſerved for the ſucceeding Tables. It has been before obſerved, that nearly 1-5th of the inſane, originally on their admiſſion, were rated as incurables, from their having been more than one year unremittingly deprived of reaſon, and whoſe proſpects of recovery will hereafter be diſtinctly calculated. The difference, therefore, in the general proſpects of cured and incurable, will depend upon whether or not we embrace in our eſtimate thoſe of the latter deſcription. But I affirm, from accurate inveſtigation of the Bedlam regiſters, that even of the patients admitted, at various intervals and ages, within ſeven months from the commencement of the malady, that the majority are invariably diſcharged amongſt the incurables; and I have not yet ſeen any authentick proofs of greater ſucceſs. Some recover after a few weeks, or months; but generally are detained one month longer, in a probationary ſtate of quarantine: ſtubborn caſes are kept one year. So that from the uſual ſlowneſs of the criſis and recovery, inſanity muſt be claſſed amongſt the chronic diſeaſes.

I am well aware that it may be diſputed, whether a conſiderable number of thoſe diſcharged as ſick and weak, and with fits and palſy, might not, with equal propriety, be added to the dead liſt, at leaſt in the general calculation. But this makes no alteration in the proportion or number of the cured; it only ſubtracts from the incurable to add to the dead liſt; and to increaſe the latter one third, or as 1 of 8 or 10, inſtead of 1 of 14, as before ſtated. The mental derangement, no doubt, adds to the mortality: numbers diſcharged, as troubled with epilepſy or palſy, muſt have fallen into theſe afflictions poſterior to their admiſſion, as they are always an exception. The inſane generally die of epileptick, convulſive, apoplectick, and paralytick ſtrokes, or of frenzy and atrophy. It is alſo obſerved, that more, comparatively, die of the inſane patients re-

cently

cently admitted, than of the ſtationary incurables. Formerly the mortality in Bedlam was ſwelled by extraneous diſeaſes, particularly the ſmall-pox and ſcurvy, both of which are now prevented. Melancholy and confinement, or ſedentary life, we know to prediſpoſe to ſcurvy; but by an increaſe of vegetable diet, this diſeaſe is now baniſhed from the mortal catalogue of Bedlam.

The ſixth Table illuſtrates the principal, occaſional, and remote cauſes of inſanity, together with the comparative proportion of cured, incurable, and dead, as influenced by each of theſe different cauſes; the proportion of relapſes; the ſubſequent probability of recovery, or at leaſt of a lucid interval or reſpite. We all know, by demonſtration and reading, that one eighth part of the blood is circulated through the brain: we know the origin and diſtribution of its ſpinal elongation, and forty pairs of nerves; its inveſting membranes, its diviſion into cavities and prominences, and its internal ſtructure to the moſt minute diſcernible filaments. But ſtill the latent prediſpoſition or frailty in the receſſes of the brain, which render ſome more than others liable to this mutiny of reaſon, on the application of remote and obvious cauſes, are totally unknown. Moſt of the proximate cauſes aſſigned by authors for madneſs, are mere hypotheſes; and of no active uſe to medicine, or to the community. The pretended diſcoveries of the anatomical knife, and the ſpecifick gravity or levity of the brain in ſcales; the inteſtine commotions and quarrels of the minute atoms of intellectual matter or ſpirit,

ſpirit, are all equally conjectural. The great decypherer and phyſiologiſt of the mental functions, Mr. Locke, has here taught us to deſpair, and to be convinced of the imperfection of our ſenſes and faculties. Literature, however, ancient and modern, abounds with romances, not only on the intellectual functions, and ſprings of ſenſe and motion, but alſo on the jaded topick of temperaments, of original organization, with the progreſſive revolutions, corporeal or mental, by time and age. The late Dr. Mead broached a propoſition, which has been implicitly tranſfuſed, on his credit, throughout ſucceeding authors: that from ſudden tranſports of joy, and the exhilirating paſſions, more were inſane than from contrary cauſes: and he quotes Bedlam as an inſtance during the year of the South-Sea ſcheme, when great fortunes were ſuddenly acquired and loſt. But on claſſing the different cauſes of inſanity in Bedlam, I perceive no examples in proof of Dr. Mead's aphoriſm, but hundreds in direct contradiction to it. To each of theſe cauſes we ſhall now devote a few remarks.

Some of the remote cauſes are complicated, as love and drink, misfortunes and drink, family and relapſes. Beſides, in many inſtances it is impoſſible to determine whether theſe are cauſes or effects of deranged intellects. Truth alſo compels us to add, that in many inſtances even the remote cauſes are conjectural, and are often reported from the ſurmiſes of the relations or friends of the inſane. In the firſt miſcellaneous and large group, misfortunes, troubles, &c. the incurable are to the cured rather more

than

than 2 to 1; and the dead about 1 of 10. From religion and methodiſm, or ſpiritual terrors, the odds againſt cure are nearly 2 to 1; and the mortality about 1 of 10. From ſudden frights the chances of cure are nearly equal; and the mortality as 1 of 12. Frantick and diſappointed love ſeems to have been a torment of both ſexes, in which the odds againſt cure are nearly 2 to 1; and the mortality about 1 of 10. The patients from drink were moſtly males, in which the odds againſt cure are about 2 to 1; the mortality as 1 of 10. Of inſanity ſoon after parturition, the proſpects of recovery are equal; and the mortality inconſiderable. From fever the chances of cure are nearly equal; but the mortality is as 1 of 8: moſt of theſe were in conſequence of fever: but at the ſame time inſanity is ſometimes a "*luſus naturæ*" of the intermittent and remittent type. From family and hereditary inſanity, the incurable are not conſiderably predominant above the cured: there are ſeveral inſtances of cure when hereditary from each of the parents: the dead are as 1 of 13. From pride there is a ſingular and monſtrous increaſe of incurables. From ſtudy the odds are more than 2 to 1 againſt cure. From venereal infection, or irregularities during the uſe of mercury, the chances of recovery are equal. Contuſion, fracture, &c. afford favourable preſages. Upon the whole, the various exaſperating and depreſſing paſſions of mind ſeem, more than all the other cauſes, to give riſe to inſanity. If to the preceding we add faults of the blood and bile, and circulation in the *vena porta*, plethora in the brain; opium chewed, or intoxicating poisons snuffed up the nose, two Asiatick practices, we shall have enumerated most of the exciting causes of this humiliating disaster; and we may also add of suicide: of which hereafter.

Relapses may be considered both as a cause, and an effect of the imbecillity. We are left by the registers to guess at the original causes of some hundreds of such cases: but reason and analogy induces us to ascribe them to some of the most universal causes before mentioned; and probably in the same proportion. They are in danger of relapses from all the preceding causes which originally give birth to insanity; but in what proportion, from each of these different causes, they are most prone to relapse, I could not, with sufficient exactness, unravel. Multitudes of the relapses are either of patients discharged, cured, from Bedlam, or of others brought there, for the first time, for admission. It must strike readers with surprize to observe, that the relapses in Bedlam are not greatly short of one half of all the patients. But on the other hand we are to reflect, that numbers of these are repetitions and re-admissions a second, a third time, or oftener, of the same patients. Another discovery is made by this Table, that in our Bedlam roll of 2,800 insane: these are not all, by some hundreds, distinct individuals, but relapses of the same patients. No disease is more prone to relapses. These are, at various intervals, in different persons, from one to upwards of twenty years; and during this period either one or many relapses. Some melancholick on relapses have only a periodical invasion of profound grief, want of sleep, inappetency, restlessness,

leſſneſs, anxiety. I am inclined to think, that on promiſcuous calculation the chances againſt relapſes into inſanity cannot be eſtimated at more than 4 to 1. In calculating the proſpects of cure, we are not to omit the dangers of ſubſequent relapſes, that is, whether the cure is palliative or radical. Medical and political reaſons render this an intereſting problem to be determined. After relapſes, and thoſe even reiterated, the prognoſticks are as favourable, and indeed more ſo than in recent attacks; almoſt one half of the relapſes again recovering: and the inconſiderable danger of death does not exceed the ordinary proſpects and blanks of life. From the proportion of cured, incurable, and relapſes, we ſee how difficult it is as yet to reſtore the intellects to their healthy tone.

The ſeventh Table demonſtrates the comparative proportion of cured, incurable, and dead, as influenced by youth and by age. This is divided into three intervals, two of the extremes, and one of the middle ſtages. The difficulties of cure are evidently progreſſive, according to the age: from 10 to 20 years of age it is 1 and ¼ to 1 in favour of cure: on the other hand, from 30 to 40 years of age it is 2 to 1 againſt cure: and from 50 to 60, 3 to 1 againſt cure. The proportion of mortality in inſanity alſo correſponds with the different ages, and in reality ſeems nearly to keep pace with the general proſpects of life, independent of the diſeaſe. Thus, under 20 years of age, only 3 *per cent.* die: between 30 and 40, 10 *per cent.*: and between 50 and 60, 12 *per cent.* die.

The

The eighth Table diſplays the comparative proportion cured of thoſe admitted into Bedlam after 1, 2, 3, 4 years, and upwards, from the firſt manifeſtation and uninterrupted perſeverance of the calamity. From the end of 12 months to 2 years, the cured are about 13 *per cent.* or 1 of 8: between 2 and 3 years, about 3 *per cent.*: 4 years is the lateſt period that I can find of any perſon recovering the perfect exercise of reaſon. By means of this Table we alſo evolve a radix, by which to aſcertain the proportion of thoſe who probably recover when diſcharged incurable from Bedlam, after 1 year's trial. And in calculations formed upon a general ſcale, and upon the Bedlam regiſters, theſe ſhould be added to the cured; and an adequate reduction ſhould be made from the incurables.

The ninth Table demonſtrates the different periods of life when inſanity, from hereditary taint, uſually burſts out. The principal interval is between 20 and 50 years of age; and both in features and event frequently differs from the lineal ſimilitude. Nor ſhould we omit to remark, that of 213, reported as inſane from family pollution, 35 of them are hereditary and relapſes combined: from whence we may preſume, that moſt of the others were the firſt eruption of the diſeaſe, although appearing ſo late in life. Whether, and in what proportion from hereditary taint relapſes are more frequent, than from other accidental cauſes, cannot be determined from the preſent regiſters. I conceive, that relapſes from hereditary contamination are here defective by at leaſt one third.

Laſtly,

Laſtly, in ſtating any caſe, or aſking any medical opinion of the proſpects of cure in inſanity, the following preliminaries are requiſite: the time elapſed from the manifeſtation of the diſeaſe, the ſymptoms, the cauſes, the age. From the preceding data, the anſwers will not be difficult; and in the calculation we are not to forget relapſes. No partial prognoſticks, in the uſual mode of deduction from traditionary ſymptoms and cauſes, can be depended upon in inſanity above all other diſeaſes in the morbid catalogue. The opinions, therefore, of medical individuals, as to the conſequence or duration of the malady, are as far inferior to medical arithmetick in aſcertaining truth or probability, as the oracles of old were to the demonſtrations of Euclid. The principal prognoſticks and data furniſhed by the ſymptoms, excluſive of thoſe already analyzed, are, that in ſome degree of mania more favourable hopes are entertained, than in fixed gloomy melancholy: inauſpicious ſymptoms are no intermiſſions or remiſſions, or lucid intervals of reaſon; indecency with reſpect to the calls of nature, frenzy, epilepſy, apoplexy, palſy, atrophy. Phyſiognomy is a theme too complicated for our preſent inquiry. In contradiction to medical doctrines, and on the authority of Mr. Gozna, neither from the ſeaſons, nor from the phaſes and changes of the moon, is the tide of frenzy in any conſiderable degree affected in Bedlam.

In concluding this ſubject I have the pleaſure to add, that Mr. Gozna did me the favour to peruſe the manuſcript before it went to the preſs, and that he coincides with me, both reſpecting the

the juſtneſs of the calculations, and the concluſions. In the group of vexatious paſſions, I left to the reader the analyſis of thoſe originating from neceſſity, avarice, ambition; their various complications, &c.

CHAP. VIII.

DISEASES of the External Senſes; including viſion, hearing, ſmell, taſte; to theſe we ſhall add the diſeaſes of the voice and ſpeech; ſterility, and morbid irritability of the generative organs. The derangement of thoſe delicate and precious ſenſes through which we derive ſuch ſupreme delight; through whoſe avenues are conveyed into man the firſt rudiments of his ideas and knowledge, are important objects of medical ſcrutiny; notwithſtanding very few from theſe cauſes are in danger of mortality. But the extent of our propoſed plan requires, that we ſhould not only include thoſe diſeaſes which deſtroy life, but thoſe likewiſe which annoy mankind. I could have wiſhed to aſcertain from regiſters, in conformity with my general plan, the proportion of cured and incurable in this group, and the average of blind; alas! I found our hoſpital records too inaccurate.

Viſion. The principal diſeaſes may be comprehended under ophthalmia, fiſtula-lachrymalis, gutta-ſerena, cataract, ſpecks on the cornea. I exclude ſome other natural defects, rather than diſeaſes, ſuch as myops, preſbyops; for the cure of which the optician is the beſt phyſician.

Ophthalmy, or inflammation of the eyes is a frequent complaint: it may be in the exterior membranes of the globe, or in the edges of the eye-lids; or may be a complication of both; it may be in one, or in both eyes; it may be general, partial, external, internal, temporary, chronic, idiopathick, ſymptomatick: of all which ſpecies there are various gradations. The external is by far the moſt frequent form of ophthalmy; and, under diſcreet management, is attended with trifling danger: ſometimes, however, it is followed by ſpecks on the cornea, or calloſity, and blindneſs. Violent inflammation has extended to the interior parts of the eyes, the choroid and retina; and if not relieved in the courſe of fourteen days, there is danger of incurable blindneſs.

Fiſtula lachrymalis. This partial inflammation affects the lachrymal ſac and ducts, and obſtructs the deſcent of the ſuperfluous moiſture of the eyes into the noſe, hence this fluid neceſſarily trickles down the cheeks, and the eye is overflowed: on preſſure of the internal angle and puncta lachrymalia, there is alſo a diſcharge of glareous ſerum, by which the eye-lids, during ſleep, are glewed together. The degrees of inflammation and obſtruction are various. In the inveterate ſtages it may terminate in abſceſs, ulcers, and caries of the contiguous naſal bone.

Gutta-ſerena, amauroſis; in one or in both eyes, and in various gradations, from obſcure viſion to cheerleſs tenebroſity. To a ſpectator the eyes appear nearly as in health, only that the pupil is dilated and inanimate; the retina insensible to the rays of light, and the iris mute, without corresponding contraction or enlargement: a physiognomist might say, there are no sensitive emanations or magnetick rays emitted through this mental mirrour. It attacks suddenly or gradually, and sometimes intermits; but in general it is chronic, and always dangerous; often irremediable.

Cataract may affect one eye, but in general both; and commonly is gradual in formation, weeks, months. It arises from disease or opacity of the crystalline lens obstructing the visual rays in their course to the retina. The consistence and colour of the lens is various, white, pearl, green, yellow; and from these the occulist forms his prognostick. In couching the eye the pearl-coloured is preferred: the white is too soft; the green and yellow incurable; as is also that species wherein the strongest rays of light excite no contraction of the pupil.

The predisposing and occasional causes of injured vision and of opthalmy, are external violence and blows; sudden suppression of perspiration; extraneous bodies or acrids admitted within the eye-lids; acrid metallic fumes, and noxious exhalations; long exposure to confined smoke, especially from wood fires; smoky houses and cottages; acrid collyria; epidemick state of the air, and infection; long continuance of wet weather; long exposure of the eyes to the rays of strong light, to snow, or luminous objects; cold streams of air; suppression of salutary evacuations, or cutaneous eruptions, and of chronick ulcers; acrimony of the blood;

blood; interruption to the free return of blood from the head; frequent intoxication; nocturnal studies; long want of sleep, grief, tears; small tubercles within the eye-lids; ulcerated eye-lids; variolous; morbillous; scrophulous; venereal; erysipelatous; rheumatick; catarrhal; intermittent; herpes; cancerous. Of fistula-lachrymalis, the causes are inflammation of the lachrymal sac, or ducts. Of gutta-serena, the causes are plethora, distention of the vessels of the retina; palsy of the optick nerves, general or partial; diseases of the brain, or of the retina; profuse and suppressed evacuations; excess of venery; chronic headach; ebriety; cachexy; venereal; intermittent; symptomatick in the irregular gout, apoplexy, &c. Of the cataract, the causes are opacity of the crystalline lens. The general causes of injured vision, exclusive of ophthalmy, may be briefly enumerated; and are long attention to minute objects; weakness of the power to contract the pupil; faults of the globe; defect of the aqueous humour, its impurity or density; opacity of the lens, or of the vitreous humour; the retina callous or too sensible; faults of the optic nerves; contraction, concretion, flaccidity of the pupil; gibbous or convex lens or too near and flat; dropsical eye; spasm, or palsy of the ocular muscles; diseases and ulcerations of the eye-lids and ciliary glands; ulcers and fistula, specks and scars in the cornea; films growing from the angle of the eye; inversion, also elongation, and concretion of the eye-lids; various diseases of the brain from internal or external causes.

Hearing, injured by deafness, noise in the ears, by inflammation and consequently excruciating

 pain:

pain: the firſt is a frequent infirmity in old age. The prognoſticks are deducible from the cauſes.

The cauſes are faults in the original ſtructure of this curious and complex organ; defect of the auricle, ſtraitneſs of the external auditory tube, its obſtruction or concretion: obſtruction, relaxation, calloſity of the tympanum by hardened wax, mucus, ſerum, ulcers, luxuriant fleſh; caries, luxation of the ſmall auditory bones; obſtruction of the veſtibule, cochlea, labrynth; laxity, dryneſs, induration of the membranes; palſy, and ſpaſm of the internal auditory muſcles; conſtriction and obſtruction of the euſtachian tube; colds, catarrh, obſtructed perſpiration, rheumatiſm, plethora, ſuppreſſed evacuations, diſorders of the ſtomach, coſtiveneſs; nervous, loud exploſions, age, fever, ſoporous diſeaſes, and diſeaſes of the auditory nerves, and of the brain; ſymptomatick in ſeveral diſeaſes.

Smelling too acute, or blunt, or unnatural. The cauſes are, the membrane lining the noſe, rigid, dry, deficiency or exceſs of its mucus, tenſe, irritable, obſtructed, ſchirrhous, callous, carious, ſtifled with polypus, ſnuff; palſy of the olfactory nerves; diſeaſes of the brain; ſordes and pus in the olfactory ſinuſſes; and alſo in the mouth, gums, teeth, tongue, larynx, fauces; foul effluvia from the ſtomach. *Sternutation* is ſymptomatick in ſeveral diſeaſes; but ſometimes, is a primary malady, and has been known to infeſt hours, days, or even weeks. The cauſes are, epidemick influence of the air; ſuppreſſed naſal hemorrhages, or cutaneous eruptions;

tions; venereal; worms, or abſceſs in the ſinuſſes; diſeaſe of the brain.

Taſte depraved. The cauſes affect the principal guſtatory organ, the tongue: and are ſordes of the tongue and mouth in various diſeaſes; the ſaliva in quantity or quality diſeaſed, and either depraved from the blood, or from waſhing over diſeaſed parts of the mouth or palate; tenſion or laxity of the guſtatory organ, or papillæ; faults of the lingual nerves; diſeaſes of the ſtomach, fauces, noſe, tongue, lips, &c.

Voice and Speech. Under it may be included hoarſe, guttural, ſtridulous, deadened, ſtifled ſound at the glottis; ſtammering, liſping, defect and impediments in articulation, muteneſs. The cauſes are, defect or waſte of mucus by exertion of the voice; deſtruction of the mucus ducts of the larynx; its cartilages oſſified; injury of the recurrent nerves; laxity and palſy of the muſcles of the glottis and contiguous cartilages; venereal; changes of weather; ſymptomatick in ſeveral diſeaſes. Voice and ſpeeeh may alſo be injured in all the various parts of their complicated organization; the larynx, pharynx, tongue, uvula, fauces, noſe, palate, gums, teeth, lips.

Sterility of the ſexes; no inconſiderable number of both ſexes are incapacitated from exerciſing that important and divine function of giving creation to their own ſpecies. The cauſes direct both to the prognoſtick and cure.

The cauſes in the male ſex are, palſy, or torpidity of the penis, or its nerves, or generative organs; the penis ſhort, monſtrous in ſize, its prepuce ſtraitened; impediments in the urethra and ſeminal ducts, teſticles, epididymis, vaſa deferentia; the ſemen inert, vapid, aqueous, ſcanty; weakneſs of the ejecting or accelerator muſcles; corpulency; too tenſe erection; old age; caſtration, manuſtupration, too frequent coition, extreme chaſtity, venereal diſeaſe, inebriety, broken conſtitution, tabes-dorſalis. In the female ſex, morbid ſtructure of ſome part of the generative machinery of the ovarium, fallopian tubes, womb, vagina, labia, clitoris; ſtraitneſs, concretion, obſtruction of the vagina or womb from inflammation, ſcirrhus, polypus; cold frigid temperament; promiſcuous coition; exceſs of venery, irritability; fluor albus, obſtructed menſes, irregular menſtruation; cachexy.

Morbid irritability of the genitals, including priapiſm, pollution, furor uterinus. Here the fabulous ſyren incantations are realized. This is the Scylla and Charybdis in which multitudes of juvenile conſtitutions and lives are wrecked; more eſpecially of the male ſex, and the pampered ranks of the community. Of involuntary pollution we have treated under dorſal tabes. In our climate the uterine mania rarely occurs in that extreme of indecency deſcribed by authors. The ſame diſeaſe has happened to ſome women who had the mortification to be linked with impotent huſbands.

The cauſes of morbid irritability of the genitals are, acrid ſerum, ſpaſm, inflammation in the urethra, vagina, or other generative organs; irritation of the bladder, womb, rectum; obſtructed menſes; fluor albus, heat, excoriation of the vagina, venereal; ſtimulating, acrid, diureticks,

diureticks, and emmenagogues; ſtimulating diet and drink, exceſs of venery, manuſtupration, libidinous books; gleets; protruſion of the vagina; habit; local, nervous, or muſcular irritability.

CHAP. IX.

DISEASES of the Stomach and Inteſtinal Tube, are very univerſal and frequent maladies in both ſexes, and throughout all orders and ages. The ſtomach and alimentary canal are furniſhed with numerous nerves; and the ſenſibility of the former very acute, eſpecially at its upper extremity. The length of the convoluted alimentary tube, from the mouth to the anus, is five or ſix times the length of the whole body: into this contractile ſewer are inceſſantly heaped food and drink, beſides a variety of copious ſecretions from the body, requiſite in the proceſs of digeſtion and aſſimilation of chyle, as ſaliva, pancreatick fluid, bile, mucus, and arterial exhalation from its internal ſurface.

Within the ſhort ſpace of a few weeks, the generality of mankind conſume more food and drink than amounts to the whole weight of their bodies. This diurnal ſuperfluity and load, together with the corrupted and abraded animal parts of the body, and the different ſecreted fluids, muſt again, in a few hours, be expelled through the principal human excretories: in the healthy ſtate, by far the ſmalleſt proportion of the alimentary ſuperfluity is through the inteſtinal or fecal excretion: the greateſt part is abſorbed by the lacteals and lymphaticks, intermixed with the blood, and afterwards filtered by urine, perſpiration, and in the puerperal ſtate, milk. But in their reſpective proportions, prodigious diverſities enſue from exerciſe or reſt, ſleep and waking, paſſions of mind, the quantity or quality of food, cleanneſs of the ſkin, conſtitution, climate, ſeaſon, atmoſphere, and the alternation with each other of theſe excretions. Again, when we reflect that from the ſmall parotid glands, between a pint and a quart of ſaliva is ſecerned during the twenty-four hours; and on the prodigious ſecretion through the kidneys, we may eaſily conceive in the natural and morbid ſtate, what a conſiderable quantity may be ſecerned from the liver, the largeſt of the abdominal viſcera: making, however, ſome deduction for the ſlower circulation through the vena porta.

The chart of London diſeaſes demand ſome criticiſm on that inextricable miſcellany Surfeits, Stoppage of the Stomach, Vomiting, Cholick and Gripes, Bloody flux. In the laſt century, ſurfeits make a monſtrous article in the chronicle of deaths, amounting in ſome years to four hundred; whereas, during fifteen years of the preſent century, they ſink down to only fifteen. Yet all are witneſſes that good eating and gormandizing are not worn out of faſhion in this metropolis. Phyſicians know that ſurfeits and intemperance are often merely prediſ-

poſing

posing or occasional causes of diseases: they may rouse latent disorders, or dispose the body to receive noxious impressions externally. The searchers therefore formerly, as I suspect, made many of these reports from the ostensible cause which they imagined gave birth to the disease and mortality. At the same time, I am not contending for the delicacy and moderation of our forefathers appetites. They were unquestionably in the last century, and partly indeed from the cheapness of flesh-meat, and scarcity of vegetable nutriment, more carnivorous in their diet than the present generation.

Stoppage of the stomach also, is a morbid centaur in the last century. It would baffle the ingenuity of an antiquarian to decypher the true import of this term: severe sickness, or the word Abracadabra, would be full as intelligible. It is a vulgar name for rejection of food; and there are few diseases in which the stomach does not sympathize. What proportion of the mortality of infants, adults, or the sexes, are crammed into this absurd article, I submit to the reader's criticism.

An important circumstance, and overlooked so far as I know, by all the calculators and criticks on the rise and fall of infant diseases in London, is this. In the first column of 15 years, at the beginning of the present century, Colick and Gripes of the guts amount to 13,668, but continue through every succeeding column to diminish; and in the last or fifth, dwindle to 769 only. What is meant by this complaint, colick and gripes? was it dysentery? We observe that bloody flux makes a separate, though small

ſmall group through all the five columns. Were theſe two diſeaſes confounded in the annual reports? or may it not be alledged, that many infant diſeaſes and deaths, which were formerly crowded into colick and gripes, are in modern times transferred to the vortex of convulſions? I am aware that, in reply, it may be ſuggeſted that drains, ſewers, drier lodgings, leſs damp, alteration in diet, and the more plentiful uſe of vegetable and fermented liquors, have decreaſed dyſenteric complaints in this city; and alſo, that Dr. Sydenham, in 1670 and 71, deſcribes an autumnal dyſentery as annually prevailing in London, and about two months in duration. Turning the ſubject into every poſſible view, I continue to ſuſpect that numbers of infant diſeaſes, and commonly terminating fatally in convulſions, were formerly heaped into gripes and colick; for during the laſt thirty years of the preceding century, they amount to the enormous number of 69,799.

Manducation. Diſeaſes of the teeth are the principal impediments to the exerciſe of this function. There are few adults who cannot deſcribe the pangs of tooth-ach from their own feelings. It is generally intermittent, and ſeldom dangerous to life, except during the firſt dentition of infancy.

The cauſes are, inflammation of the perioſtium of the teeth, gums, or jaws; ſuppreſſed perſpiration; moiſt air; catarrhal defluxion; ſuppreſſed habitual evacuations, naſal hemorrhage or veneſection; plethora; intermittent; ſcorbutick; arthritick; rheumatick; caries of the teeth; ſugar eat; beetle and tobacco chewed;

ed; acrimony of the blood or ſaliva; ſpirituous liquors; mercury; ſuppuration in the maxillary ſinuſſes and gums; ſpungineſs and flaccidity of the gums and perioſtium; irritation and diſorder of the fifth pair of nerves; nervous ſympathy.

Deglutition interrupted. We very ſeldom meet with this ſimilitude of Tantalus, wherein food or drink is either ſwallowed with difficulty and pain, or totally interrupted in its deſcent to the ſtomach, and regurgitated by the mouth and noſe. The cauſes lead to the prognoſticks.

The cauſes are, ſpaſmodick conſtriction of the œſophagus, and in various parts of that tube; palſy of the muſcles of deglutition; tumours, polypus, or ſcirrhus in the pharynx, œſophagus, pylorus, trachea, thyroid or dorſal glands; aneuriſm and enlargement of the aorta; ulcers in the œſophagus; luxation of the os hyoides; compreſſion of the pharyngeal nerves; cachexy, worms, crudity; extraneous ſubſtances ſtuck in the throat, ſymptomatick in angina.

Diſeaſes of the Stomach are, idiopathick and ſymptomatick. Under the preſent head we ſhall include inappetency, indigeſtion, nauſea, vomiting, eructation, acidity, cardialgy, heartburn, regurgitation of bile, pica, bulimy, or water braſh, ſoda, pyroſis, hiccup, rumination. Several of theſe are obvious ſymptoms, and are often complicated. Chronic diſeaſes of the ſtomach, and other organs ſubſervient to digeſtion, and aſſimilation of chyle, eſpecially the liver, are frequent maladies; they are the forerunners and cauſes of many diſeaſed and ſhattered conſtitutions; and are more frequent amongſt pampered mortals than amongſt the indigent and induſtrious

The prediſpoſing and occaſional cauſes of all the preceding diſeaſes of the ſtomach are in general, weakneſs of its muſcular coats; diſeaſes of its nerves; ſmall omentum; the digeſtive menſtrua, as bile, ſaliva, mucus, defective or depraved; frequent exſpuition and waſte of ſaliva; ſlow digeſtion, and corruption of food in the ſtomach; crudities in the ſtomach; vitiated chyle; exceſs of pituita, acidity, bile; relaxed pylorus, large ſtomach; calculi in the biliary ducts; ſcirrhous ſtomach; pancreas, liver, ſpleen, duodenum; abraſion of the mucus of the ſtomach; ulcers, cancer, depreſſion of the xiphoid cartilage; frequent emeticks and purgatives; valetudinarian regimen, too much phyſick, quackery, and care about health; gluttony, epicuriſm, pampered indulgence of that paſſion and appetite; frequent ſurfeits, dram-drinking; exceſs in malt liquors; the aliment in quantity or quality, or in multiplicity at one meal, injurious; adulterations of fermented or diſtilled liquors; unwholeſome waters; ravenous ingurgitation at meals, and imperfect manducation; fat, rancid, corrupted, ſalted, and indigeſtible farinaceous food; tea, tobacco, watery liquids. In infancy, acid milk, ſucking to exceſs, curdled milk in the ſtomach; ſuperfluous acid generated in the ſtomach; too violent agitation in the nurſe's arms; paſſions of the nurſe; too tight bandages; exceſs of ſaliva ſwallowed during dentition; too much vegetable diet and milk. To the catalogue of general cauſes may be added various depreſſing and cankering paſſions of mind; cares and troubles; want of

ſleep

ſleep, intemperate ſtudy, ſedentary life, unremitting application to ſedentary buſineſs; moiſt cold air, foul air of cities; leaning forward on the ſtomach, and improper poſtures of the body; coſtiveneſs; ſuppreſſion of ſalutary evacuations and cutaneous exanthemata; ſanguineous plethora; hereditary infirmity, bad health, old age, chloroſis, worms, gout, rheumatiſm, intermittent and remittent fevers, and various other acute and chronic diſeaſes; poiſons; extraneous ſubſtances ſwallowed, contuſions on the head; external injuries; blows and falls.

Cholera Morbus is much more frequent in tropical and warm climates; and in northern regions in the ſummer and autumnal ſeaſons, eſpecially in unuſually hot ſummers. The diſeaſe is not unfrequent in this iſland and metropolis; nor is it entirely reſtricted to the warm ſeaſon only. The nauſea, ſickneſs, vomiting, and purging, either commence about the ſame time, or alternate with each other: and throughout its rapid race there is ſeldom any fever; it is often a ſalutary effort of nature, by which a ſuperfluity of bile is diſembogued; and in caſes of ordinary violence, may continue a day or two, and then ceaſe. In more tremendous aſſaults, with ſinking of the vital powers, it ſometimes proves fatal in twenty-four hours.

The prediſpoſing and occaſional cauſes of cholera morbus are, hot climate and ſeaſons; in warm climates extreme heat and dry weather, ſucceeded by a fall of rain and coolneſs of the atmoſphere; ſudden changes of weather; increaſed ſecretion of bile and corrupted bile; ſurfeits, intemperance, accumulation of feculence

lence in the inteſtines and liver; exceſs of food or drink without ſufficient exerciſe; indolence, luxurious living and ſedentary life; malt liquors; paſſions of mind; repulſion of cutaneous eruptions; gout; poiſons; worms; ſymptomatick in intermittent and remittent fevers.

Dyſentery, bloody flux, ſpurious remittent. Of its abatement in London we have already ſpoken at the beginning of this chapter. This debilitating, painful, and contagious diſeaſe, has been before mentioned, under remitting and autumnal fevers. It is called by Sydenham and Morton, the ſpurious remittent, and fever of the ſeaſon, turned on the inteſtines; of which it is a complication and degeneracy; there exciting frequent ſlimy, often bloody ſtools, with ſevere ſickneſs, cholick, gripes, and urgency to exonerate the inteſtines. When fatal, many are deſtroyed between the ſeventh and twentieth days, by gangrene, or if later, by lientery or dropſy. I have ſeen medical records where only 1 of 20 died.

The cauſes of dyſentery are, warm climates and ſeaſons, marſhy effluvia; cold nights followed by warm days; ſudden ſuppreſſion of perſpiration, eſpecially in warm climates; expoſure to cold and moiſt air and rains, and wet cloaths and beds; long continuance of ſultry and dry weather; exceſs and corruption of bile; ſymptomatick; dyſenterick contagion from privies, beds, &c. relapſes from irregularities or intemperance.

Diarrhœa, flux, temporary and chronic, including the celiaca, lienteria, morbus hepaticus, niger, atrabilis. In the ſimple diarrhœa, the evacuation by the anus is unnaturally frequent

frequent and liquid, accompanied with gripes, but not ſo excruciating as in the dyſentery, with inappetency, dry ſkin, thirſt, hectic, but no conſiderable fever; nor is it contagious. In the ſeverity and evacuations there are varieties, and in ſome caſes it is ſalutary; when not chronic, nor with emaciation or cachexy: to infants it is frequently pernicious. In the celiaca the aliments and chyle are ejected: in the lienteria, like a bucket whirling into a well, food is no ſooner taken than diſcharged. The morbus hepaticus is without pain or teneſmus, with dark flux of blood and ſerum, or like ink; and both in colour and conſiſtence various.

The cauſes of diarrhœa are, exceſs of food and drink, or acrid putreſcent aliment; new fermented liquors; unwholeſome waters uſed in aliment; vegetable laxative food; feculence, ſtercorous, pituitous, bilious, in the inteſtines; vitiated digeſtion, with morbid irritability of the inteſtinal tube; irritability of this muſcular canal, and increaſe of its periſtaltic motion, atonia; exceſs and acrimony of bile, warm climates, broken conſtitutions, cachexy, chronic dyſentery, immoderate flux of humours to the inteſtinal tube, and exhalation by the arterial extremities of that canal; ſuppreſſion of perſpiration, and of other evacuations; ſuperfluity of ſerous humous; impediments in the abſorption and paſſages of the chyle; obſtruction in the vena portarum; laxity of the pylorus; palſy of the ſphincter ani; ulcers ventricular or hepatic, repelled gout, and raſh; ſudden paſſions of mind; nervous irritation; eroſion or rupture of the blood-veſſels on the interior ſurface; obſtruction

of

of the ſpleen; acrid diſſolution of the blood; colliquative; worms; ſymptomatick in fevers; purgatives; poiſons; habit. In infancy, acidity; dentition, exceſs of ſaliva or milk ſwallowed; corrupted milk and chyle, thin laxative vegetable diet; errors of the nurſe in diet; gravel in the kidneys.

Coſtiveneſs, it is true, is frequently ſymptomatick in many diſeaſes, but it is alſo idiopathick; and the ſuppreſſion of this excretory, during ſeveral days, occaſions vertigo, headach, diſturbed ſleep, inappetency, indigeſtion, flatulence, colick, &c.

The cauſes of coſtiveneſs are, obſtruction or conſtriction of the inteſtinal tube; faults in its muſcular fibres; diminution of irritability by age or diſeaſe; defect of mucus and of bile, eſpecially cyſtic bile, or its inertneſs; coſtive food, drink, or medicines; too little drink; exceſſive diſcharge by perſpiration or urine; indolence and hard feces; particular ſituation and air; habit.

Colick. We here aſſociate together the inflammatory, ſpaſmodick, ſaturnine, bilious, flatulent, the infantile colick, and other ſpecies. From ſlight or ſerious attacks of this torture few of the community are exempted. Colick is generally a temporary diſeaſe; with which ſome, much more than others, are afflicted at intervals. Inflammation of the inteſtines, ileus, volvulus, enteritis, has been confounded, and often fatally, with inflammation, or with nephritick paroxiſms in the kidneys and ureters, which are hereafter diſcriminated. Inteſtinal inflammation is ſometimes alſo the effect and not the original cauſe

cauſe of colick. It is always extremely dan gerous and precipitate; frequently deſtroying in a few days, ſometimes in one day, and is ſeldom protracted beyond nine. There is leſs danger in young than in old perſons: unfavourable ſymptoms are, unconquerable coſtiveneſs, immoderate vomiting, tumid abdomen, eructation, hiccup, cold extremities, gangrene.

Under the ſpaſmodic colick may be claſſed the colica pictonum, ſaturnina, plumbeia, and dry belly-ach of the Weſt Indies. This writhing pain in the abdomen, attended with obſtinate coſtiveneſs and retraction of the navel towards the ſpine, infeſts various claſſes of artificers; ſometimes terminating in chronic colick, in palſy of the lower extremities, and in convulſions.

Bilious colick is accompanied with ſevere pain in the ſtomach and inteſtines, nauſea, bitter taſte, ſickneſs, vomiting of bile, coſtiveneſs, anxiety, dejection of ſpirits. Its duration is ſhort, but it is prone to return on any intemperance or irregularity; ſometimes it ends in jaundice.

Flatulent colick is diſtinguiſhed by the pain being mobile, without much nauſea or vomiting, or hard pulſe or thirſt, or fever; by conſiderable unuſual diſtention of the abdomen, and flatulent exploſion upwards and downwards; and more or leſs interruption of reſpiration.

The infant colick is very frequent, and infinitely more fatal in thoſe years than the London bills repreſent. It is variouſly complicated with vomiting, coſtiveneſs, or diarrhœa: infants often ſcream lamentably, and cannot be appeaſed.

N The

The predifpofing and occafional caufes of colick, inflammatory, fpafmodick, bilious, and of moft other fpecies are, acrid matter of aliment, medicines, poifons; acrid putrid bile: obftruction of the inteftinal tube by indurated feculence, hair-balls, cherry-ftones, calculi, fteatome, hydatides, intufefception, contraction of the inteftines in fome part; fcirrhus, cancer; fevere colick, fpafm; ruptures; wounds of the inteftines; the aliments, pickles, condiments, and luxuries of the table, cooked, prepared, or preferved in lead, or copper veffels not well tinned; the lead corroded from clayed veffels ufed for domeftick purpofes; wine adulterated with lead; cyder preffed in leaden cifterns; effluvia of lead to which painters and fome metallurgifts are expofed; excefs or acrimony of bile; broken conftitutions in tropical climates; abrafion of the inteftinal mucus; acrid chyle; particular food or drink; new fermented liquors; intemperance; fudden fuppreffion of perfpiration; cold wet feet: fudden paffions of mind; inteftinal flatulence and elaftic air; mufcular and nervous fpafms; plethora menftrual, lacteal, hemorrhoidal; fcorbutick, rheumatick, arthritick, hyfterick, nephritick; calculi in the biliary ducts; epidemick; aneurifm of the aorta; turgid gall-bladder; fpafm in the abdominal mufcles, violent vomiting; habitual, hereditary. In infancy, corrupted meconium, crudity, and four or adulterated milk; fuction to excefs; acrid bile; the mother or nurfe fafting too long before the infant fucks; corrupted unwholefome milk of nurfes; nurfes addicted to paffion, to dram-drinking; infufficient exercife of the infant;

fant; tight rollers round its abdomen; too long continuance of vegetable nutriment; dentition; worms.

Gall-Stones, calculi cyſtici. We have no account of this diſeaſe in ancient records. Until the beginning of the preſent century, it had eſcaped the vigilance of medical obſervation. But it is now known, that biliary concretions are, perhaps, not leſs frequent than thoſe in the urinary organs. Gall-ſtones infeſt more the adult, old, and ſedentary; and it is alledged, more females, as is the caſe in jaundice, than males. In attempting to deſcend through the gall-ducts, they excite direful pain at the ſtomach and hepatick region, and often a jaundice colour; but, at the ſame time, without any acceleration of the pulſe and circulation. In the expulſion of the calculi, there are uſually reiterated exacerbations and remiſſions of pain. The continuance of the paroxiſms is from a few hours to days, weeks, or even months; but the latter is rare; during which period either no ſtone is diſcharged, or one or many ſtones are ſucceſſively protruded. The calculi vary in ſize, ſhape, colour, conſiſtence, and numbers; from a pea to a walnut, and from one to dozens and ſcores. It is generally a tedious and chronic diſeaſe, but is ſeldom immediately dangerous, unleſs, as in nephritis, inflammation is kindled, or during pregnancy. When chronic and inveterate, it may terminate in jaundice, cachexy, dropſy. The cauſes are, hereditary, viſcid, tenacious bile, ſedentary life, depreſſing paſſions, ſpirituous liquors; often ambiguous.

Jaundice, icterus, morbus regius. Some of the eaſtern nations have naturally this ſallow complexion, both of the ſkin and eyes. The mortality by jaundice in the London bills, during the laſt thirty years of the preſent century, amounts to 2169; and in the preceding century is doubled.

Of 70,000 patients admitted into the Alderſgate Diſpenſary, from 1770 to 1788, and which, as I have frequently mentioned, is acceſſible to all ages and diſeaſes, thoſe afflicted with jaundice were only 162: and of theſe the males were 66; the females 96; and their ſundry ages were as follow:

Ages.		Numbers.
Under 10	——	13
From 10 to 20	——	5
20 to 30	——	41
30 to 40	——	36
40 to 50	——	36
50 to 60	——	14
60 to 70 and upwards		17
Total	—	162

Of theſe cured 114—Dead 9—Relieved 9—Diſcharged 31

From this Table it is manifeſt, that jaundice is neither a frequent nor formidable diſeaſe, at leaſt in this metropolis and iſland: that one third more of females than males are afflicted with it: that it is more frequent after 20 than before that age in the proportion of 9 to 1: that more than two of every three are certainly cured. The relieved, diſcharged, or not accounted for, are a dubious and neutral liſt, the majority

majority of which may be added to the incurable and dead.

The generick ſymptoms of jaundice are, a preternatural ſaffron tinge of the eyes, ſkin, and urine; inappetency, indigeſtion, and coſtiveneſs. It may be critical, ſymptomatick, idiopathick, periodick, chronick, and ſometimes, though very rarely, is local. From gall-ſtones it is generally periodical; and ſuch are prone to relapſes. The prognoſticks are more favourable with natural ſweats; in recent than in chronic; in youth than in old age; in robuſt than in weak perſons; in yellow than mulatto tinge; and when not complicated with other dangerous diſeaſes, eſpecially dropſy. Its duration and termination is various; from a few days to weeks, and months.

The prediſpoſing and occaſional cauſes of jaundice are, ſand, mucus, or inſpiſſated bile in the biliary ducts, eſpecially the ductus communis; tumors compreſſing the biliary ducts, or their concretion; ſcirrhous duodenum; ſpaſmodick, and flatulent colick obſtructing the inteſtinal orifice of the biliary ducts; violent paſſions of mind; ſtrong emeticks or purgatives; ſudden refrigeration of the body; hepatic obſtruction and inflammation; languid circulation through the vena porta, ſedentary life; warm climates and broken conſtitutions; exceſs of bile and re-abſorption; cachexy; depraved ſtate of the blood; ſymptomatick in ſome intermittent and remittent fevers, pregnancy, ſcurvy, obſtructed ſpleen; venomous bites and ſtings. In infants, exceſs of bile and meconium, or diſtention of the duodenum obſtructing the biliary excretory.

Worms. In aſſigning an adequate ſhare of mortality to worms, the London bills, probably, are defective. During the laſt thirty years of the preceding century, they are rated at only 1400; and continue decreaſing throughout the preſent century. Perhaps a portion of verminous mortality is confounded with colick and gripes, or with hectic emaciation. Worms infeſt moſt in infancy and childhood; but ſeldom until after ablactation; and then, probably, more of the children of the neceſſitous than of the affluent. The principal ſpecies of human worms are the rotunda, or lumbricalis, the tænia or lata, the cucurbitina, and the minute aſcarides; theſe are again, but with ſuperfluous ſubtility, ſubdivided by noſologiſts. Worms differ in ſhape, in length, in the different portions of the inteſtinal canal in which they burrow; and in the different periods of life in which each is moſt troubleſome to the human ſpecies. Verminous ſymptoms are numerous, various and extremely ambiguous, unleſs worms are diſcharged with the feces; feculence in the ſtomach and inteſtines may occaſion all the other ſymptoms. But without a ſymptomatick fever, children purſue their uſual amuſements, and are rarely confined to bed.

The cauſes of worms are, improper diet for theſe years, as cheeſe, farinaceous, legumens, fruits, ſaccharine, putrid diet or unwholeſome aliment, hereditary weak conſtitution, moiſt air: the ova of the inſects ſwallowed with the air, food, or drink, often ambiguous.

Hemor-

Hemorrhoides, piles. Is a frequent and very univerſal diſeaſe in both ſexes, and moſt ſo during the adult ſtages and decline of life; and by which the lives of many are incommoded and harraſſed. They are diſtinguiſhed into the blind or imperforated lumps and tumors about the margin of the anus; and into open or bleeding piles; into external and internal; and are temporary, periodical, and chronic. Sometimes the tumours and hemorrhage from the anus enſue without any previous diſeaſe of the body; but generally ſome antecedent or accompanying diſorder is felt, and eſpecially ſymptoms of plethora, either general or local. The quantity of ſanguineous extravaſation is various in different perſons, and in the ſame perſon at different periods: but is rarely immediately fatal. Theſe imperforated tumours, and ſanguinous torrents, are almoſt always periodical, and at various intervals. They are often ſalutary, if moderate, eſpecially if bad health preceded; and alſo as preſervatives. For in the decline of life, when the hemorrhoidal flux has been frequent, but ſuddenly ceaſes, they are in danger of apoplexy or palſy. On the other hand, in exceſs, it may exhauſt the body, injure the health, and terminate in dropſy or conſumption. Or ſometimes hemorrhoidal tumours inflame, ſuppurate, and form fiſtulas in ano.

The prediſpoſing and occaſional cauſes of piles are, hereditary; plethora, ſizy blood, luxurious living, indolence and ſtimulating diet; intemperance, eſpecially in ſpirituous liquors; dried indigeſtible diet; ſuppreſſion of the menſes, and their final ceſſation, and of other critical evacuations; obſtructions of the liver, ſpleen, of the meſenteric and hemorrhoidal veins; reiterated and ſevere colick; abraſion of the inteſtinal mucus; acrid purges; acrimony of the blood; coſtiveneſs, coſtive habit, and hardened feces; worms; ſitting too long on the neceſſary, and over-warm ſteams, or ſtoves; long ſitting, riding, and compreſſion of the hemorrhoidal veins; gravel in the kidneys or ureters; diſeaſes of the vagina, womb, and neck of the bladder; prolapſus ani; pregnancy; rupture of the extremeties of the iliac arteries; effuſion of blood into the cellular texture of the inteſtines, near the extremity of the rectum; habit.

Vomiting of Blood, hematomoſis, vomitus cruentus, is a very rare diſeaſe. It is ſaid to be more frequent in females than males; and is an adult malady: the colour depends upon the time it has lain in the ſtomach, and is with intermixtures of food, bile, pituita: there is alſo great proſtration of ſtrength, and proneneſs to faint. The quantity of this extravaſation is various, from ounces to pounds; and frequently ſome portion deſcends by the anus. It is extremely dangerous, either immediately, or in its conſequences. If with fever and great force in the diſcharge, it may deſtroy in a few paroxiſms; or if chronic, may end in dropſy, conſumption, or diſeaſes of the ſtomach and inteſtines. Slight eruptions have relieved chronic maladies of the liver and ſpleen, hypochondriaſm, hyſtericks, and intermittents. From obſtructed menſes it is much leſs alarming.

The cauſes of vomiting of blood are, obſtructions of the liver, ſpleen, menſes, hemorrhoides;

rhoides; ſcirrhus of the ſtomach and liver, or ſpleen; ſuppreſſion of habitual diſcharges or evacuations, or old ulcers; dregs of intermittent fevers; ſcorbutick; acrids and poiſons ſwallowed, and violent efforts to vomit; worms; violent paſſions; external injuries.

Poiſons. By poiſons conveyed through the mouth or wounds, very few of the community are deſtroyed, at leaſt accidentally. The ancient Aſiaticks, Greeks, and Romans, were infected with the ſilly infatuation and apprehenſion of conſtantly ſwallowing poiſon in their aliment. This was not an epidemical error of the rabble, but had ſpread amongſt their emperors and philoſophers: hence the pompous and abſurd compoſitions of mithridate, theriac, and other poiſonous antidotes. None of the two hundred genera of the quadruped creation, nor of birds, are poiſonous; and very few of the fiſh, or of the numerous inſects and reptiles. Out of the many thouſand genera of the vegetable creation, the poiſonous are comparatively trifling: ſuch are the napelli, apocyna, ſtrammonium, ſolanum, laurus, aconitum, manchinel, cicuta, opium, and a few others; ſome of which, however, are powerful remedies. Of the mineral, the metals and ſemi-metals, arſenick excepted, the preparations of lead, copper, and mercury, are alſo amongſt the potent remedies.

Of poiſons, ſome corrode or burn, others are ſeptic; and by far the greateſt number attack the vital principle, by either violent irritation or torpidity: ſome have a more deadly malignity than others, and are more ſpeedily deſtructive. Moſt of the vegetable poiſons excite narcotic, ſtupifying, vertiginous, lethargic, convulſive, and emetic ſymptoms, affecting the brain, external ſenſes, heart, and ſtomach. The minerals, as arſenick and corroſive ſublimate, excite ſymptoms of inflammation in the ſtomach, in the moſt violent degree; and both copper and lead of ſpaſmodic colick alſo. From their readier ſolution in the ſtomach, the vegetable poiſons, except by the ſymptoms, can rarely be ſubjected to ocular detection; but by certain chymical analyſis, or by the ſmell, when in any conſiderable quantity, the mineral may be diſcovered. Theſe obſervations, and many of thoſe relating to inſanity, are a part of medical juriſprudence: and we ſhall hereafter touch upon it, under female abortion, and external violence, eſpecially injuries of the head.

Hydrophobia. Phrenitis latrans, rabies canina, aquæ fugax. There are very few inſtances of this diſeaſe in Britain: it is, notwithſtanding, one of the modern hobgoblins, in which we rival the folly of the ancients reſpecting alimentary poiſons. It ſhould firſt be indiſputably aſcertained whether the dog, or other animal, was mad or not: we have a thouſand falſe alarms, forgeries, and falſehoods in this reſpect. Dogs, eſpecially puppies, are ſubject to periodical ſhort fits, in which they run about as if mad, barking inceſſantly, and with a querulous angry voice. It is agreed, that canine madneſs is more general in hot climates, and in the hotteſt ſummers of northern. But unfortunately hitherto, in moſt caſes, probably nineteen out of twenty, the mania of dogs has not been incontro-

incontroverbly decided; as in cafes even at the commencement, when it is very dubious, dogs are very impoliticklv deftroyed, inftead of being confined in a place of fecurity, to obferve whether the poifon is fermenting in them. Hence, probably, much ideal terror and horror; and boafted, though impotent, virtues of many vulgar noftrums, panaceas, and antidotes.

In the human fpecies, confirmed hydrophobia, or excruciating difficulty, pain, horror, and convulfion, in attempting to fwallow, efpecially fluids, is defcribed as invading fome weeks, and even months after the venomous bite or wound: and the exacerbation to be influenced by the lunar phafes and changes. There are fome inftances of recovery in thefe laft and defperate ftages. For my own part, I will not deny the probability of fome fpecifick poifon being conveyed by fuch bites and wounds: but many reafons incline me to believe, that hydrophobia has often been miftaken for tetanus: and fome cafes, perhaps, might be afcribed to ftrong imagination and terror. The difeafes from other venomous bites and ftings are transferred to the future clafs of external accidents.

CHAP.

CHAP. X.

DISEASES of the Urinary Organs. During the laſt 30 years of the preceding century, thoſe marked in the mortal catalogue of London as cut of the ſtone, gravel, and ſtrangury, are only 1796; and at preſent the mortality is more inconſiderable; and perhaps, in ſome degree, may be accounted for by modern improvements in the cure of the venereal diſeaſe, and in the operation of lithotomy; for as to lithontripticks, we are as yet ignorant as of the philoſopher's ſtone. From Dr. Dobſon's Treatiſe it appears, that out of 192,394 ſick of various diſeaſes, medical and ſurgical, in different county hoſpitals, throughout England, 430 of theſe underwent the operation of lithotomy. Some countries, more than others, are obnoxious to calculous concretions; which have been variouſly imputed to air, food, drink, and water. Gravel and ſand in the urinary organs is a frequent complaint, to which infancy and childhood are by no means ſuch martyrs as adults, thoſe eſpecially in the decline of life: but from the ſhortneſs and width of the female urethra, they are preſerved freer from calculi in the bladder than the male ſex. Diſeaſes of the urinary organs have been often deſcribed by authors under three general heads: Iſchury means a total ſuppreſſion of urine; and from the ſeat of the diſeaſe is called renalis, uretoria, veſicalis: Dyſury is only a ſlighter degree of the former:

mer: Strangury, a conſtant irritation to urine, and in ſmall quantity, with heat and pain.

Inflammation and Calculi of the Kidneys, nephritis, nephralgia; and generally confined to one kidney. The ſymptoms, fever, acute pain and heat in the lumbar region, varying in ſeverity and torture; frequent efforts to micturition, and the urine in ſmall quantity, red, bloody, ſabulous; ſometimes total ſuppreſſion, with vomiting, colick, coſtiveneſs. The rheumatick lumbago, with which, as I before obſerved, it may be confounded, is a very different diſeaſe. It is always dangerous and precipitate, eſpecially when the urine is ſuppreſſed, terminating within ſeven, or, at the utmoſt, fourteen days, by diſcuſſion, ſuppuration, gangrene, ſcirrhus.

But the moſt frequent malady about the fountain of the urinary ſecretion, is from Calculi in the ureters. The kidneys have few nerves, and therefore not very acute ſenſation. Calculi or gravel in the ſtrainers of the kidneys, ſeldom excite much uneaſineſs until they are forced into the ureters by the current of urine, by exerciſe, exertion and agitation of the body, paſſions of mind, ſtimulating diet and drink: then they excite atrocious pain, which is exaſperated by certain poſtures, by every motion of the body, and by a full ſtomach; together with all the other ſymptoms common to inflammation, except the fever; to which, however, and to inflammation calculi often give birth. At the beginning the urine is limpid; afterwards it becomes turbid and ſabulous. This is a chronic diſeaſe, and too frequently with intermiſſions, nephritic exacerbations, and relapſes, at uncertain

tain intervals: and by thofe who are not thoroughly verfed in morbid prognofticks, may be confounded with inteftinal colick.

Inflammation and alfo Calculus of the Bladder. Of cyftitis, the fymptoms are acute burning pain in the region of the bladder and perineum, and extending to the loins; tumour, tenfion, and hardnefs of the lower part of the abdomen from the diftended bladder, perpetual painful efforts to urine and ftool, and the former either fuppreffed, or in fmall quantity. It is very rapid and dangerous: total fuppreffion within a very few days excites burning fever, lethargy, delirium, convulfions, gangrene: or even after recovery from a violent difeafe, incontinence of urine may remain for a confiderable time.

Of calculus, or ftone in the bladder, the fymptoms are all dubious, without founding with the furgical inftrument. It is a chronic difeafe, flow in accumulation; and is frequently endured many years, without having recourfe to lithotomy. The fymptoms vary in feverity, and recur in exacerbations at uncertain intervals; fuch are frequent irritation to urine, and difficulty in the evacuation, and fometimes fudden ftoppage; ftrangury, tenefmus. The fize, fhape, and number of ftones are various: often only one, but fometimes feveral are extracted by lithotomy.

Inflammation and obftruction of the urethra cannot be thoroughly inveftigated, without a defcription of the venereal difeafe, to which we have not yet arrived.

The

The predifpofing and occafional caufes of urinary fuppreffion, obftruction, and ftrangury, whether originating in the kidneys, ureters, bladder, or urethra, are inflammation of the kidney or ureter, calculi or fand in the kidneys or ureters; acrid diureticks; fpirituous liquors; plethora, fpafm, poifons, fevere riding, violent heat and mufcular exercife; ftrains of the lumbar and dorfal mufcles; long continuance in a bent or fupine pofture; inactive fedentary life; wounds, contufions, abfcefs; defecation and crifis of other difeafes by the kidneys; fcirrhous, incyfted, dropfical, paralytick kidney; gout; inflammation of the bladder or its fphincter, ftone in the bladder; too long retention of the urine, by which the bladder becomes violently ftretched, and paralytic; hernia of the bladder; obftructions in the neck of the bladder, or in the urethra; varicous blood veffels; fcirrhous, or enlargement of the proftrate glands or feminal veficles; inflammation, caruncles, and ftricture in the urethra; thicknefs of the corpus cavernofum; contiguous difeafes of the anus, vagina, and womb; hardened feces, hemorrhoides, wounds of the rectum, fiftula; ulcers of the womb, obftructed menfes, or their retention in the vagina; pregnancy; ulcers and worms in the kidneys, bladder, or urethra, and excretion of acrid pus or membranes, by urine; grumous, extravafated blood in the bladder and urethra; infpiffated femen after coition; excefs of venery; too acute fenfibility of the urethra, defect of mucus; acrid urine; tartarous and aftringent wine or drink, food, or medicines; ftimulating food and drink; frequent ebriety;

ebriety; terreſtrious water; ſudden refrigeration of the body; contuſion; old age; plethora; lunar, venereal, rheumatick, arthritick, hyſterick, ſcorbutick, dropſy, violent colick, retraction and ſhrinking of the penis.

Incontinence of Urine, and alſo Diabetes. Of incontinence, or eneureſis, authors make three ſpecies, one involuntary, without ſenſe or effort, which is often rebellious to remedies; the ſecond involuntary, but with a knowledge of its excretion; the third involuntary, during ſleep only. The Diabetes was unnoticed in the London bills until the preſent century; and perhaps its trifling depradations were thrown amongſt conſumptions. It denotes a chronic diſcharge of urine beyond the natural quantity, and ſometimes exceeding in weight all the fluids and ſolids taken by aliment: it is generally clear and colourleſs, but ſometimes white and chylous, or unctuous, or, like honey diſſolved in water, and taſtes ſweet: there is unquenchable thirſt, intenſe heat, ſlow hectic and emaciation, pain in the loins. It often invades by ſlow and imperceptible ſteps, and without any other diſorder, until, by long continuance, emaciation is viſible, with debility and obſcure fever. It is ſometimes periodical, and in hyſtericks ſymptomatic.

The prediſpoſing and occaſional cauſes of incontinence of urine, involuntary, are, palſy of the ſphincter of the bladder, from either too great dilatation and accumulation of urine, or from violent efforts in parturition; debility, old age; exceſs of venery; fiſtula, abſceſs, ulcers, lithotomy, ſtone, ſpaſm, gout, apoplexy, palſy,

external

external injuries. Copious, acrid urine; irritability of the bladder from inflammation, ulcers, excoriation, defect of mucus; ſpaſm, relaxation of the ſphincter; weakneſs of the ſphincter ani, and accelerator muſcles; pregnancy, laborious parturition; compreſſion and irritation of the bladder; habit.—Of diabetes the cauſes are, aqueous tenuity, and alſo acrimony of the blood; weakneſs, laxity of the kidneys and renal veſſels; imperfect coheſion of the craſſamentum of the blood with the ſerum; faults in the aſſimilation of the nutriment, and ſanguification; exceſs of watery drink and ebriety; diureticks; ſudden refrigeration of the body, and ſuppreſſion of perſpiration; unuſual determination of blood and ſerum to the kidneys; exceſs of venery; increaſe of cutaneous abſorption; obſtructions of the abdominal viſcera; ſpaſm; nervous; habit: often unknown.

Ulcers in the Kidneys and Bladder, and Bloody Urine. The ſymptoms of ulcers in the kidneys are, thick fetid urine, ſometimes with mouldered fragments of the kidneys; heat and weight in the loins; hectic emaciation, ſtupor of the leg, and ſome other ſymptoms of nephritis, It is tedious and dangerous. Of ulcer in the bladder the ſymptoms are, pain in the pelvis and perineum, exaſperated at intervals; heat, ſtrangury, dyſury; the urine fetid with intermixtures of pus, mucus, and blood; ſometimes the rectum alſo is eroded. Of bloody urine, or hematuria from the kidneys, ureters, bladder, ſeminal veſicles, or urethra; from the kidneys the hemorrhage is ſometimes profuſe, and the blood of various colours, according to its ſolution and ſtagnation in the bladder; the urine tinges linnen dipped into it of a red colour, and the extravaſated blood is coagulable by heat. There are inſtances of its periodical flow, like the menſes.

The prediſpoſing and occaſional cauſes of urinary hemorrhage are the general cauſes of hemorrhages; calculi in the kidneys or bladder; falls, blows on the loins; violent exertion of the lumbar muſcles, riding, exerciſe; venery; plethora; obſtructed evacuations, hemorrhoids, menſes; hemorrhoids of the bladder and varicous veins; acrid diureticks; ulcers; ſymptomatick in ſcurvy, putrid ſmall-pox, and malignant fever.

CHAP. XI.

DROPSY. During the laſt thirty years of the preceding century, dropſy and tympany in London amount to 23,366. In the preſent century, dropſy makes about one *twentieth* ſhare of the London funerals; and annually in Europe amounts to 200,000: and is one of the oligarchy of morbid tyrants. It has been alledged, that more women die of this internal deluge than men; and, according to Sydenham, more of the former at the final menſtrual ebb, than at any other period. But

ſo

ſo far as my reading extends; neither its proportion to other diſeaſes; neither the age or ſex in which it is moſt predominant; neither the mortality abſolute or comparative; nor the proportion of cured and incurable have to this day been decided from facts or numbers. I therefore, through my learned friend, Dr. Sims, procured the regiſters of diſeaſes in the Alderſgate Diſpenſary of London, which is acceſſible to all ages and diſeaſes, and to both ſexes: the reſult of this ſcrutiny is as follows:

A TABLE, demonſtrating the comparative proportion of dropſy to other diſeaſes in London: the proportion of males and females afflicted with this diſeaſe: the ages or ſtages of life when dropſy is moſt predominant: the proportion of cured, relieved, diſcharged, and dead, in this diſeaſe; founded upon the regiſters of the Alderſgate Diſpenſary, from 1770 to 1788.

Of 70,000 patients, dropſies, were	1,188
Dropſical males 439; dropſical females	749

The ſundry ages of thoſe dropſical were:

Comparative ages.		Numbers.
From birth to 10 years	———	106
10 to 20	———	53
20 to 30	———	112
30 to 40	———	249
40 to 50	———	323
50 to 60	———	209
60 to 70	———	110
70 to 80	———	23
80 to 90	———	9
Total	———	1188

Cured.	Relieved.	Diſcharged, or not accounted for.	Dead.
674	56	275	186

Theſe

These include every genus and species of dropsy, the hydrocephalus and hydrocele; neither of which were numerous: and the former principally fatal to children under ten years of age. Anasarca was the most frequent genus; and next to that, Ascites. Besides, all cases of anasarca and œdematous legs were ranged amongst this dropsical group; nor was it possible to form an estimate of the genera separately, as the word Hydrops was often indefinitely used.

From these data we may draw the following conclusions: That dropsy is in the proportion of one 70th to all other diseases: that it is more inimical to the female than to the male sex: but at the same time it must be recollected, that in London, and other cities, the women are considerably more numerous; which somewhat detracts from the comparative excess in them of dropsical mortality. That dropsical ravages are principally amongst adults: for notwithstanding that one half of the community are under twenty years of age, yet but a small portion of these are dropsical. It is chiefly against adults, and those in the decline of life, that dropsy prowls with slow and sullen destruction; and is as 8 to 1 more general after twenty, than before that period. For reasons, which physicians of experience will anticipate, we may add to the dropsical dead list some of the relieved, discharged, and not accounted for. It appears, therefore, that, under skilful medical treatment, rather more than one half of dropsies, promiscuously, were cured; that about one third or fourth died; that of those afflicted with dropsy of the brain, lungs, or abdomen, the majority are,

are, as yet, incurable. The proportion of cures and deaths, in conſequence of the radical or palliative operation of the hydrocele, I could not yet procure materials to aſcertain.

Dropſy in the Brain and Spine, hydrocephalus, and ſpina bifida, is moſt frequent in infancy and childhood; but is often very difficult to detect, and the ſymptoms at the beginning are dubious. Theſe are, fixed pain, lethargy, obſcure viſion, inappetency, decay of ſtrength. It is commonly ſlow in increaſe; from months to a year, or more. It is ſeldom cured; and the fatal termination frequently palſy and convulſions. Sometimes it is complicated with the ſpinal dropſy.

Dropſy of the Thorax, hydrops pectoris, and pericardii: in one or both ſacs of the pleura, or in the pericardium; or in the pulmonic cellular texture. This is much leſs frequent than the abdominal; and is often very difficult in the early ſtages to be detected; as the ſame, or nearly ſimilar ſymptoms, occur in ſome other obſtinate diſeaſes of the breaſt and lungs. Sometimes it is circumſcribed and local; at other times, it begins by anaſarca, and is complicated with univerſal dropſy of the other cavities, or with aſthma; ſometimes it conſiſts of hydatides. It is diſtinguiſhable from the empyema, and from the polypus and aneuriſm of the large veſſels, by the ſymptoms peculiar to each. After ſome fevers, thoracic dropſy has formed with ſurprizing rapidity. The fatal event is often preceded by hemoptoe, anxiety, and accelerated reſpiration.

The dropſy of the pericardium muſt neceſſarily clog the functions of the lungs, and much more the motion of the heart, and circulation of the blood. But from ſimilarity of ſymptoms it may be confounded with ſome other pulmonick diſeaſes.

Abdominal Dropſy, including the aſcites, the dropſy of the ovaria, fallopian tubes, and womb. The aſcites, or exudation between the peritoneum, inteſtines, and viſcera, is much more frequent than the hydrothorax. In ordinary caſes it is diſtinguiſhed by the preternatural enlargement and prominence of the abdomen, ſenſe of fluctuation to the fingers and ears, ſcarcity of urine, thirſt, coſtiveneſs, ſqualid countenance: and where the accumulation of water is conſiderable, the functions of reſpiration are incommoded; eſpecially in a horizontal poſture. It may occur either ſingly, or as a part of univerſal dropſy. The ſerous tranſudation is the general form of aſcites; but ſometimes it is of a gelatinous conſiſtence, and more of coagulable lymph from the blood, and the fluctuation not perceptible: in other caſes it is incloſed in numerous morbid cyſts, called hydatides; which may be ſuſpected, but cannot be known to a certainty, until after the experiment of tapping. Some ſurvive many years under aſcites, and after reiterated evacuations by tapping; on the whole, often amounting to ſeveral hogſheads of water. In others, there are inſtances of accumulation ſo extraordinary, ſudden, and profuſe, as to render it neceſſary to be drawn off repeatedly in the ſhort interval of a few weeks. Aſcites encyſted; from broken conſtitutions;

conſtitutions; unſound viſcera; the conſequence of other diſeaſes; chronic; with decay of appetite; emaciation, hectick, teazing cough; with urine conſiderably diſproportioned to the drink, with inceſſant thirſt, purple livid ſpots, general debility, lethargy, are all ſpecies unfavourable, ſome deſperate.

Dropſy of the ovaria, fallopian tubes, and womb, are female, and not unfrequent maladies. It is rarely that both ovaria or tubes are affected at the ſame time. The diſeaſe begins with a ſoft tumour at one ſide of the abdomen, generally increaſing by ſlow gradations, and at length ſometimes to an enormous ſize and weight, accompanied with ſeveral aſcitic ſymptoms, but the fluctuation is imperceptible, or obſcure; and the extravaſation is often encyſted and gelatinous. Both are too often incurable. Dropſy of the womb is a very rare diſeaſe: it has been deſcribed as occurring either in the pregnant or unimpregnated ſtate; and in the latter caſe, as contained within the cavity of the womb, or between the fetal membranes and the womb; or within the layers of the membranes.

Dropſy of the Cellular Membrane, externally, under the ſkin; including anaſarca, leucophlegmatia, œdema. It generally appears firſt in the lower extremities, and there too only in the evening, diſappearing by a horizontal poſture in the night: at length aſcends, progreſſively, to the legs, thighs, trunk, and ſcrotum; and in ſome inſtances, to the face, particularly in the mornings. The intumeſcence of the ſkin is pale and ſoft, and, on the preſſure of the finger, indents; but is ſoon again filled up with

 water.

water. As it increaſes to a univerſal anaſarca, there is difficulty of breathing, particularly after exerciſe, ſcanty urine, thirſt, decay of ſtrength, ſlow hectic, diminution of the natural heat. Sometimes the legs and thighs only are enlarged and diſtended to a monſtrous magnitude; their ſkin burſts, ulcerates, or is irritated to eryſipelatous inflammation. It is either complicated with aſcites or hydrothorax, or beginning as œdema, and increaſing to anaſarca, it oozes through all the external cellular texture; and having inundated all theſe cells, proceeds in drowning the vital organs.

Dropſy of the Scrotum, hydrocele. This is a local diſeaſe, confined to the male ſex; and to which all ages are ſubject. There are two principal ſpecies; that between the vaginal coat and teſticle, and that in the ſpermatick chord; and either collected in cyſts, or diſperſed through all the cellular membranes incloſing the ſpermatick veſſels. In general, hydrocele is confined to one teſticle, at the beginning is not painful, and neither diminiſhes nor diſappears, nor is capable of reduction into the abdomen; nor is accompanied with the uſual alarming ſymptoms of protruded inteſtinal rupture. Hydrocele has not only been miſtaken for inteſtinal rupture, but alſo for ſcirrhous teſticle, and venereal induration. Beſides, ſcrotal hydrocele and hernia, hydrocele and ſcirrhous teſticle, hydrocele and encyſted dropſy of the ſpermatick chord, have been ſeen combined. Some hydroceles are ſeveral years collecting: others are very ſuddenly formed, eſpecially from extravaſated blood, external injuries, violent muſcular exer-

 tions;

tions; theſe likewiſe have been miſtaken for ruptures. Hydroceles vary in the quantity of fluid and magnitude, containing from ounces to ſeveral quarts; ſome are enormous in ſize, occaſioning great load, and pain in the back. In the preternatural thickneſs of the ſurrounding ſkin and membranes, and alſo in the colour of the extravaſated fluid there is great variation. Many, from choice or neceſſity, not chuſing to riſk what is termed the radical operation and cure, are contented to drag on life merely by frequent repetitions of the ſcrotal puncture or palliative remedy.

The prediſpoſing and occaſional cauſes of dropſies, comprehending all the preceding genera, are various acute and chronick diſtempers; broken conſtitutions, cachexy; intermittent, remittent, and ſcarlet fevers; repelled eryſipelas; rickets; jaundice; biliary obſtructions; ſuppreſſion or repulſion of habitual or wholeſome evacuations, as menſes, hemorrhoides; general debility from various cauſes; atony of the ſanguinous veſſels, and of the exhalents, and tranſudation of ſerum through them; exceſſive evacuations by hemorrhage, diarrhœa, perſpiration, or other excretories; ſudden and large draughts of cold water when the body is much heated, eſpecially if not diſcharged by urine or ſweat; exceſs of fluids, of ſpirituous liquors; languid circulation; ſedentary life; watery trades; moiſt air; ſuppreſſed perſpiration, and watery excretions; tenuity or impurity of the blood; tenacious adheſion and agglutination of the coagulable lymph; increaſe of ſerous fluid in the blood; diſeaſes and alſo ruptures

tures of the lacteals and lymphaticks, and of the kidneys, ureters, and bladder; defect of lymphatick abſorption; obſtructed and ſcirrhous viſcera, meſentery and lungs; aſthma, polypi, oſſified arteries, exceſſive fatneſs, and other cauſes intercepting the circulation of the blood: diſeaſes of the ſtomach and digeſtive organs, and thoſe of ſanguification; laxity of the external ſubcutaneous cellular membrane; debility of the muſcular ſolids and fibres, and of the tela celluloſa; hereditary; hydatides; violent muſcular exertions, external injuries.

Tympany. Of this diſeaſe there are two ſpecies; that where air is confined within the inteſtinal tube; the other, where it is extravaſated between the inteſtines and peritoneum: this laſt ſpecies very rarely occurs, and only from an eroſion of the inteſtines. The ſymptoms of tympanites are, chronick tumour and diſtenſion of the abdomen, compared to the ſtretched head of a drum, without fluctuation or thirſt; and not altered by the change of poſture, with inappetency, indigeſtion, colick pains, eructation, and exploſion of fetid air by the mouth and anus; coſtiveneſs, ſallow complexion; difficulty in breathing; emaciation, hectic, and atrophy. Its increaſe is generally quicker than aſcites; it is alſo chronick, and contumacious to medicine.

The cauſes of tympanites are, atony and palſy of the inteſtinal tube; exceſſive purging; chronick colick, dyſentery and diarrhœa, or their premature ſuppreſſion; ſuppreſſion of the lochia or menſes; the conſequence of rickets, intermittent fevers, aſthma, hypochondriaſis;

diſeaſed

diſeaſed abdominal viſcera; exceſs of pituita, or bile; complicated with aſcites, and the inteſtinal tube debilitated by ſoaking in water.

Exceſs of Fat, obeſitas, polyſarcia; including anaſarcous obeſity, abdominal corpulency, and their complication. This is a frequent malady of adult age in this iſland; and either in its immediate or ſecondary effects, is too often the cauſe of abridging the ſhort term of exiſtence. It ſeldom occurs before the human body has ceaſed to grow taller. The cauſes are, hereditary; laxity of the cellular membrane, or tela celluloſa; eſculent luxuries, ſenſual living, epicuriſm, malt liquors, exceſs of oleaginous ſecretion from the blood.

CHAP. XII.

FEMALE Diſeaſes, including obſtructio-menſium, chloroſis, profluvium menſium, fluor albus, hyſteria. Theſe derangements of the human machinery, which, from the days of Hippocrates, have been diſcriminated by ſpecifick morbid names, are notwithſtanding unnoticed in the London regiſters; unleſs perhaps riſing of the lights, ſpleen, and vapours are ſubſtituted as a portion of hyſterick mortality. The fatal tranſitions of the others are probably buried in conſumptions and dropſy. This formidable

midable phalanx, whoſe frequency and fatality are of univerſal notoriety, muſt be muſtered amongſt the chronic hoſt of diſeaſes. From about the period of puberty, ſeldom earlier, they begin to infeſt numbers of the female ſex. On a careful peruſal of nearly one half of the books of the Alderſgate Diſpenſary in London, and before mentioned, during ſix years, I found the total ſick and diſeaſed amounted to 29,511: by far the greater proportion of which were adults, and more females than males. Of this twenty-nine thouſand, the numbers afflicted with different female complaints were as follow: Obſtruct. menſ. and chloroſis, 254; profluvium menſ. 270; fluor albus, 446; hyſteria, 1104; total, 2074.

Here it is worthy of obſervation, that four only of the principal female infirmities conſtituted one 15th part of all the diſeaſes in that diſpenſary, which is open to afflicted patients of every deſcription and age. I ſhould, however, not omit to add, from the information of one of the learned phyſicians of that charity, that under fluor albus, a few caſes of venereal gonorrhœa were concealed; and that under hyſteria, were arranged all female and nervous complaints, without ſtrictly attending to its generick ſymptoms. We have here likewiſe, one proof that uterine relaxation is a more frequent female malady than obſtruction, in London: it is more ſo in warm than in cold climates: and probably, all theſe four female diſeaſes are more prevalent amongſt the higher and luxurious ranks; and in city than in country.

Hippocrates

Hippocrates has truly ſaid, "Uterus ſexcentarum œrumnarum mulieri auctor merito dicatur." Great and important changes enſue at puberty amongſt the two ſexes, eſpecially the female, affecting their future health. In both, the organs of generation are then evolved, and the ſexes firſt capable of procreation. That periodical diſcharge of red blood from the female womb, called menſes, the index of womanhood, begins in this iſland to ooze monthly, from 3 to 5 days, and from 4 to 12 ounces, about the age of 14, 15, or 16: but its firſt eruption and final ceſſation, as well as its periodical returns, are ſometimes extremely variable. In warm climates, the menſtrual commencement is earlier, and more profuſe. The quantity of blood evacuated, the duration, the intervals, periodical returns and effects, are irregular and various; and are diverſified by climates, ſeaſons, conſtitutions, modes of life, habits, ages, and by numerous other accidental circumſtances. In different women the menſtrual intervals are from 2 to 6 weeks, or longer; but when ſtrictly regular, or the woman not pregnant, every lunar month. The firſt periods of menſtruation, and the final ceſſation by age, are two very important epochs in female life, on which much of their ſucceeding health and longevity will hinge. But, without entailing diſeaſes, many women are liable to ſome menſtrual irregularity, with reſpect to the periods, duration, and quantity. We may add, that during the greateſt part of pregnancy, and ſuckling, the menſes do not naturally flow.

Morbid

Morbid and Irregular Menſtruation, under the different heads of ſcantineſs, chloroſis, or morbus virginius, retention, partial obſtruction, and total ſuppreſſion. The menſtrual eruption is generally and naturally preceded by heat of the loins, and weight about the uterine region, frequently with pain and cholick, laſſitude, head-ach, dulneſs of viſion, diſturbed ſleep, inappetency, and nauſea, pain and load about the breaſt: all which, with many other troubleſome ſymptoms, uſually diſappear on the eſtabliſhment of this ſalutary and critical evacuation. But where the menſes do not flow at puberty, or afterwards become obſtructed or ſuppreſſed, a numerous train of morbid ſymptoms and fatal diſeaſes often enſue; ſuch as inappetency, indigeſtion, colick, palpitation of the heart, dyſpnœa, pulmonary conſumption, hectic, dropſy, fluor albus, low ſpirits, fainting, hyſtericks, inſanity, apoplexy, cachexy, barrenneſs.

The Chloroſis appears about puberty, ſometimes indeed earlier, and alſo conſiderably later; and is more frequent amongſt indolent and luxurious females. The complexion and lips are pale, ſallow, of a green ſickly tinge; with averſion to motion, debility, inappetency, indigeſtion, craving for unuſual and unnatural food, flatulence, palpitation of the heart, laborious and quick reſpiration on exerciſe or aſcending any eminence; pain and weight about the loins, night ſweats, hectic and emaciation, œdematous ancles, uſually obſtructed menſes, unuſual bad health, and derangement of the animal, vital, and natural functions. It is ſeldom immediately dangerous

dangerous to life, but often lays the foundation of some of those diseases above enumerated.

The predisposing and occasional causes of scanty menstruation, obstruction, and suppression, and of chlorosis, may be comprehended under the following: general bad health, debility, and unsound constitutions; partial weakness of the uterine vessels; too great resistance and rigidity of the uterine vessels; want of sufficient momentum in the sanguineous circulation; scarcity of florid blood; insufficient motion and exercise of the body; sanguine plethora; sizy blood; spasmodick constriction of the uterine vessels; sudden passions of mind, especially the depressing passions; cold wet feet; cold liquors and various cooling luxuries drank or eat at the menstrual period; crude watery diet; worms; celibacy; love; salacity stifled; lax fibre; severe parturition, and local diseases inherent in the womb and vagina.

Uterine Relaxation, including excessive menstruation, fluor albus, leucorrhœa. There is a great similarity in all their causes. We here treat of menstrual excess in the unimpregnated state. Menstruation may be morbid from frequency in the returns, from suddenness of the torrent, from duration, and from quantity. It has already been said, that the quantity of the menstrual flux, the recurrence, and the duration, vary in different women: the immoderate discharge is determined not altogether by the absolute quantity, but by the morbid effects and derangement of health. Menstruation in excess, especially if chronick, is often accompanied with fluor albus; and may terminate in consumption

conſumption and dropſy, and in many of the diſeaſes enumerated, under obſtruction and ſuppreſſion; or it may prove fatal from the violence and duration of the hemorrhage.

The Fluor Albus often ſucceeds or accompanies exceſſive menſtruation. It is a dripping diſcharge from the womb and vagina, and from the ſame veſſels which exude the menſes, ſometimes pale and ſerous, or often variouſly intermixed with yellow, green, and red tinges; ſometimes fetid and acrid, and either conſtant or irregularly intermittent. At the commencement, the uſual concomitant ſymptoms aſcribed to this diſeaſe, ſuch as pain and weakneſs in the back and loins, inappetency, indigeſtion, pale ſickly colour, &c. only occur when the diſcharge is exceſſive, or long continued. Women of various ages after puberty, married and unmarried, ſome even after the final menſtrual ceſſation, are obnoxious to this gleet, which is not, as in venereal gleet, infectious. The fatal termination may be in ſome of the different diſeaſes conſequent of obſtructed and exceſſive menſtruation; ſuch as barrenneſs, diſeaſes of the womb; colick, piles, ſtrangury, hyſtericks, low ſpirits, conſumption, dropſy.

The prediſpoſing and occaſional cauſes of exceſſive menſtruation and of fluor albus, are, many of the general cauſes of hemorrhages, already enumerated; plethora, ſedentary, luxurious life, ſtimulating and nutritious diet; too long indulgence in warm ſoft beds; warm chambers; ſuppreſſion of uſual and habitual evacuations; weakneſs and laxity of the uterine veſſels from abortion, violent evulſion of the placenta,

or

or other injuries during parturition; difficult and lingering, and alſo frequent parturition; general relaxation, and delicate conſtitution; weak nerves; violent exerciſe, eſpecially in hot climates and weather; exceſſive heat of the ſeaſon or climate; moiſt watery climate; violent efforts of the body or muſcles, or ſtraining of the body and loins; external injuries, or falls near the uterine region; exceſs of venery and ſalacity, manuſtupration; ſpirituous liquors and drunkenneſs, intemperance, immoderate uſe of tea, and other warm fluids; immoderate uſe of warm baths or ſtoves; neglect of cleanlineſs and abſterſion; paſſions of mind, frights; impeded perſpiration; exceſs of ſerum in the blood; ſcorbutic habit and acrimony; purulent tranſlation to and depoſition upon the womb from other parts of the body; polypus, fungus, ſcirrhus, cancer, ulcer in the womb or vagina; procidentia uteri et vaginæ, emmenagogue medicines.

Final Ceſſation of Menſtruation from years. This is a dangerous period to women; more ſo, perhaps, than any other ſtage of maturity. The longer or ſhorter duration of menſtruation depends, in ſome degree, on its earlier or later commencement. In this iſland the menſes uſually ceaſe about 48, 45, or ſometimes at 41, and earlier; eſpecially after frequent parturition. The ſprings of life, or generative powers in females, then become effete. Towards the final drain, women commonly are irregular in the recurrence, duration, or quantity of the diſcharge; which is often exceſſive. Women who never had children, nor enjoyed ſound health;

those whose constitutions have been impaired by frequent parturition and miscarriages, and others of delicate nerves and structure, all these are frequently obnoxious to complaints and diseases at the final uterine ebb. As infirmities and bad health are frequently removed on the first flow of the menses, such are also again prone to relapse in this autumn of life, into nervous complaints, hystericks, consumption, dropsy.

Hystericks, uterine suffocation, and female nervous diseases. This morbid proteus rarely attacks before puberty, most frequently between puberty and middle age. Married and single women are obnoxious to it; but more so the latter and widows, and those barren, or irregular in menstruation. It is not so frequent amongst the laborious class, or those of clumsy organs, as in the higher ranks, and particularly in those constitutions strung to a morbid extreme of nervous and muscular sensibility and irritability. It does however affect females of robust constitutions. It very rarely attacks the male sex: the only disease in them, somewhat analogous to it, is hypochondriasm. The regular paroxism attacks generally by surprize, with a sensation of a ball ascending tumultuously from the abdomen to the glottis, and there exciting a sense of strangulation; and deviating variously into palpitation of the heart, fainting, stupor, sighing, sobbing, tears, laughter, convulsions.

The form, duration, violence, recurrence, and repetition of the hysterick paroxisms are various, not only in different women, but even in the same at different times; and, however alarming

ing in appearance, are ſeldom immediately dangerous to life: but by continuance, may derange the machine, and lay the foundation of diſeaſes. They ſometimes occaſion ſymptoms of dyſpepſy; but oftener the appetite and digeſtion are unimpaired. The prolifick brood of what may be termed nervous ſymptoms, or irregular hyſterick paroxiſms, are a medley of afflictions, and in their turn interrupt and diſturb moſt of the important functions and organs of the human body; the animal ſpirits, brain, and nerves; the heart, blood veſſels, circulation, and reſpiration; the ſtomach and inteſtines.

The prediſpoſing and occaſional cauſes of hyſtericks are, exceſſive delicacy, ſenſibility, and irritability of the nervous and muſcular fibres, and laxity of the muſcular ſolids; retention and ſuppreſſion of uſual evacuations, eſpecially the menſes; ſcantineſs and alſo exceſs in menſtruation; fluor albus; profuſe hemorrhages, and other evacuations by ſtool and urine; ſanguineous plethora; hereditary; obſtructions in ſome of the abdominal viſcera, or in the circulation of the vena porta; ſcirrhous abdominal viſcera; flatulence in the ſtomach and inteſtines; tough phlegm and ſordes in the ſtomach and inteſtines; weak ſtomach; worms; improper food; drunkenneſs; indolent, luxurious, voluptuous, ſedentary life; valetudinarian regimen; irritability of mind; paſſions of mind, particularly the diſagreeable and depreſſing, as cares, grief, diſappointed love, jealouſy, frights, intenſe fixed mental application to one object, religion, envy, anger, grievous misfortunes, joy, concealed uneaſineſs of mind; celibacy; ſalacity; ſudden

 and

and great changes in the conſtitution from menſtruation, generation, pregnancy, and parturition; impure blood; its acrid tenuity; repulſion of cutaneous eruptions; general bad health, and diſeaſed ſtate of the fluids or ſolids; irregular gout. It is often difficult and impracticable to dive into the real efficient cauſes.

CHAP. XIII.

CHILDBED Mortality in London is nearly one *eightieth* part of the whole funeral catalogue. It is in ſtorms and hurricanes; or within a very ſhort ſpace of time. The mortality of this group muſt occur between the two extremes of 16 and 50 years of age. Or, as marriages in this iſland, one with another, are computed to commence on the ſide of the woman at 25, we may, with ſafety, rate the principal puerperal mortality in the ſtages of life between 20 and 50. Of the 4½ million of annual births in Europe, excluſive of abortions, upwards of 52,000 of theſe women die annually from childbearing. On this intereſting ſubject there are ſeveral curious and uſeful propoſitions, which I have attempted to eſtabliſh by demonſtrative proof. Theſe are, 1ſt, The number of women who, on an average, die in childbed: 2dly, The proportion between natural, laborious,

rious, preternatural, and complex labours: 3dly, The number of abortive and ſtillborn infants to thoſe brought forth alive: 4thly, The proportion of twins and tergemini to ſingle births: 5thly, The arithmetical ratio and fatality of labours, and of all other diſeaſes and accidents during the puerperal ſtate.

From twenty-four years of the London, and from ſeveral country regiſters in England and Germany. Dr. Short calculates, that on an average, 1 of every 60 women die in childbed: others rate the decrement at 1 of 66, or 3 in 200. Upon a much broader baſis I formed a puerperal eſtimate. From the year 1700 to 1776, the chriſtenings in the London regiſters amount to 1,220,656; and the abortives and ſtillborn in the ſame interval, to 46,831. The ſum total therefore of the births, including the chriſtenings and the abortives, amount to 1,267,487. During the above period of 76 years, the deaths in childbed are 17,057; which number employed as a dividend to the former, makes about 1 of 74 pregnant women to periſh in childbed. But as a conſiderable number of infants, or chriſoms, after being brought into the world alive, die in the threſhold, or at leaſt before baptiſm, and conſequently are excluded from the publick enrolment of births and chriſtenings; ſeveral of them, perhaps, are ſuperadded to the abortives in the ſtrict ſenſe.

Reſpecting the proportion of natural, laborious, and preternatural parturition, Dr. Smellie ſays, "That of 1000 women in childbed, "920 of them will be delivered in the ordinary "way, with little or no accocheur trouble, ſkill, "or affiftance: 70 more of the thoufand will "be difficult labours, or flow and tedious, when "often fome fkill and aid of the accocheur will "be neceffary; and the remaining ten of the "thoufand will be preternatural labours." There will, therefore, according to this author, be about 8 *per cent.* of flow, laborious, preternatural, and anomalous labours, which, in different gradations, will be more tedious, difficult, and dangerous, than in the ufual procefs of nature.

It is a propofition not uninterefting in Obftetricks, and in medical jurifprudence, and in many inftances it is material to the obftetrical character, when unjuftly afperfed, to obferve, that, in the preceding lift, during feventy-five years in London, there were brought forth alive and chriftened, 1,220,656; that the abortives and ftillborn in the fame period were, 46,831, or as 1 of 26 to the living births. Were we, however, to add the abortions and mifcarriages of diminutive embryos, in the early months of pregnancy, and which are much more frequent than in the latter months, the abortive catalogue would be prodigioufly fwelled. Exclufive of the 4½ million of births, annually, in Europe, the abortives and ftillborn, at or very near maturity, amount to upwards of 130,000; and without including the far greater multitudes who perifh in the embryo and chryfalis ftate.

Dr. Short attempted to afcertain the proportion between fingle births, twins, and tergemini, from a regifter of three large parifhes, during a feries of years, in which the fingle births amounted ed to 11,415; the twins and tergemini to 311, or about 1 of 35.

Laſtly, Let us examine what were the ſeveral diſeaſes during pregnancy and parturition, and afterwards which occaſioned this childbed and fetal mortality, and in what arithmetical ratio were their fatality.

Of *Parturition natural, laborious, preternatural, complex,* or *anomalous.* Nine ſolar months, or thirty-nine weeks, or 273 days, reckoning from the time of conception, is the uſual period of uterine geſtation in the human ſpecies. Labour or parturition is then a ſalutary effort of nature, to expel the contents of the womb by its own muſcular contraction, and the collateral aſſiſtance of the muſcles of the abdomen, diaphragm, thorax, back, and extremities. Theſe exertions commence at intervals, called paroxiſms, or labour pains; which are various in ſtrength and duration, from one to ſeveral minutes, and recur at irregular intervals of one minute, an hour, or more.

Natural labours are all thoſe in which the infant's head preſents at the orifice of the womb; which are probably *ninty-nine* out of every *hundred* labours. But in this preſentation of the infant, ſome labours are natural and eaſy, and a ſmall number lingering, laborious, and difficult. Preternatural labours are either all thoſe wherein any other part of the fœtus ſpontaneouſly preſents at the orifice of the womb, or where, notwithſtanding the natural preſentation of the head, yet it is neceſſary to turn the infant by force, and to deliver it by the feet foremoſt. Complex and anomalous labours are thoſe, whether natural or preternatural, accompanied with extraordinary ſymptoms and danger, ſuch as floodings, convulſions, plurality of fœtuſes, &c.

Natural labours are generally terminated within a few hours, from 2 to 24 of real labour efforts; ſometimes in a few minutes, and with inconſiderable exertion or pain. Every labour in which the proceſs is prolonged beyond 24 hours, may be claſſed under the head of laborious, lingering, and difficult parturition, notwithſtanding the natural preſentation of the infant. Sometimes the labour may continue ſeveral days, but with intervals of reſpite and reſt, either from the head not entering the pelvis, or, which is much more frequent, from ſome impediment during its deſcent through that oſſious cavity. In ſome caſes, tedious and difficult labours may continue two, three, and even four days and nights, when, after reiterated paroxiſms, the infant may at length be excluded by the efforts of nature alone: in ſome of theſe caſes alſo, the mother's recovery is ſurpriſingly expeditious, as if ſhe had been delivered in half the time; and unleſs ſome dangerous ſymptoms indicate, no manual and much leſs inſtrumental aſſiſtance will be neceſſary.

The danger of the mother, from tedious and difficult parturition, is diſcernible from her natural conſtitution, her debility, pulſe, reſpiration, voice, countenance, the duration of the labour, the weakneſs of the pains, or their perſeverance and ſeverity, the ſpace elapſed from the entrance of the head into the pelvis, and from the rupture of the membranes. The danger of the fœtus may be predicted from the time

time its head has been preſſed into the pelvis, and the violence of that preſſure, eſpecially on the yielding cranial bones.

Preternatural labours are theſe wherein any other parts but the infant's head preſent at the orifice of the womb; ſuch as the feet, breech, ſhoulders, arms, and ſo on; beſides thoſe other caſes in which, although the fœtal preſentation may be natural, yet, for variety of reaſons, and in dangerous emergencies, it is neceſſary to turn the infant in utero, and to extract it by the feet. In ſome preternatural preſentations delivery may be eaſy; but in general they are always precarious, often tedious and troubleſome to the mother and accocheur; and dangerous to the infant.

Anomalous or complex labours are either natural, or preternatural; but at the ſame time are accompanied with two or more fœtuſes, or with uterine hemorrhages, or with convulſions; and to theſe ſome add the caſes of inſtrumental delivery. It is natural and uſual for the human ſpecies, and for all large animals, to bring forth one at a birth: twins often occur: tergemini are rare: four, or at leaſt five, are not ſeen in ſome millions of births. Plurality of fœtuſes are ſeldom attended with peculiar circumſtances of danger. Twins do not occaſion much difficulty; they are generally ſmall, and the remaining fœtus is ſeldom detected before the excluſion of the firſt, by which the paſſage is dilated.

Infants in the womb, we may preſume, are ſubject to diſeaſes as well as caſualties; but probably the moſt frequent cauſes of mature abortives and ſtillborn, originate from the effects and accidents

accidents conſequent upon laborious, preternatural, and complex parturition; which caſes, as we obſerved, may be eſtimated at about *eight per cent.*: but the abortives and ſtillborn are not *three per cent.* and therefore about one third only, at a medium, of difficult labours, of every denomination, are fatal to infants. In a pelvis not two inches wide at the brim, it is impoſſible for the fœtus, in whatever preſentation, to deſcend alive through ſuch a narrow paſſage. Some pelviſes have been ſeen not altogether one inch in diameter either above or below: but, happily, ſuch inſtances of deformity very rarely occur. We have but eight examples on record during the laſt hundred years in this iſland, three of them in London, and five in Edinburgh, wherein it was thought neceſſary to have recourſe to the dreadful alternative of the Ceſarian operation; and all theſe women died. During the above long interval of time, including three generations, of fifty or ſixty puerperal women in London, whoſe pelviſes were remarkably ſmall and deformed, notwithſtanding the unavoidable neceſſity of recurring to obſtetrical inſtruments, in order to diminiſh and tear away the infant, yet not above five or ſix died.

The prediſponent and occaſional cauſes of difficult, laborious, lingering, preternatural, and complex parturition, are, on the part of the Mother, ricketty formation, and deformity of the pelvis; and the common protuberance is at the jetting forward of the lower lumbar vertibra, or of the os ſacrum: the pelvis may alſo be too ſmall, without any deformity or projection; it may be too narrow from the fore to the back part,

part, above and below, and at the ſides: rigidity of the os coxcygis; too great reſiſtance and rigidity of the uterine orifice, which is a frequent cauſe; rigidity of the vagina and ſurrounding ſoft parts; firſt child; the mother in years, or long intervals between parturition; the womb too much diſtended and ſtretched, its irregular contraction, oblique poſition; the membranes too ſoon ruptured by nature or art, and the womb contracting cloſely before the infant's ſhoulders; the membranes rigid; the mouth of the womb ſtrait, callous, inert, irritable; its ſpaſmodic conſtriction; the bladder diſtended with urine; hardened feces collected in the rectum; piles; weakneſs of the mother; tedious labour and fatigue; paſſions of mind; terror and fear of the event; the mind and ſpirits broken, irritable; the mother delicate, fat, torpid, plethoric; diarrhœa, profuſe evacuations, floodings, convulſions; heat, cordials, ſtrong liquors; improper fatigue and torment, and officious endeavours in the accocheur to expedite delivery: pendulous abdomen; tumors and cicatrices blocking up the vagina; rupture of the womb; ſtone in the bladder. From the Fœtus erroneous in poſition, and different to the natural; in laborious caſes with the head either detained at the brim, or after its deſcent into the pelvis: ſuch poſtures are vertebral, occipital, auricular, mental, oral, facial. Alſo its preternatural and croſs poſitions and preſentations, the neck, breaſt, ſhoulders, arms, hands, back, loins. buttocks, breech, ſides, belly, knees, feet. The fœtus monſtrous in ſize, or only in particular parts ſuch as the head, ſhoulders,

belly;

belly; the head dropſical; the cranial bones oſſified, and not yielding in its deſcent: the fœtus dead, and blown up with putrid air: the navel ſtring twiſted round its neck; two or more fœtuſes entangled; twins growing together; deformed monſters.

Having now finiſhed the various proceſſes of parturition, with the perils and difficulties that encompaſs our immediate exit from the ſhell, I ſhall return back to pregnancy, to explore the different inconveniences and maladies that enſue in conſequence of that ſtate, both before and after parturition: many of theſe are merely temporary morbid ſymptoms; ſome of them rarely occur; others are attended with trifling danger; and a few only with imminent hazard. We may include all theſe troubleſome ſymptoms, accidents, and diſeaſes, under the following heads; proceeding progreſſively from the beginning of conception to the end of parturition, with all its train of evils.

Theſe are nauſea, indigeſtion, vomiting, pains in the ſtomach, acidity, unuſual cravings, head-ach, vertigo, coſtiveneſs, difficulty and incontinence of urine, piles, varix, pains in the back and loins, cramp, colick, fainting, œdematous legs and thighs, difficulty and labour in breathing, retroverted womb, extra uterine conception, ſuperfœtation, graviditas perennis, moles and falſe conceptions, rupture of the womb, protruſion or too low deſcent of the womb or vagina: miſcarriage and abortion, dead fœtus, uterine hemorrhage, convulſions, irregularity of the lochia, including obſtruction, ſuppreſſion or exceſs, inflammation of the womb, puerperal fever, ſever, milk fever, weed, inflammation of the breaſts, exceſs and defect of milk, inſanity.

The cauſes of many of theſe complaints during the early and latter months of pregnancy, and affecting the ſpirits, head, thorax, ſtomach, inteſtines, rectum, bladder, and circulation, originate from ſympathetic effects of conception and pregnancy; from plethora, from the bulk, weight, preſſure, and irritation of the enlarged womb, and from its ſtretching, &c.; and either ſpontaneouſly, or by proper advice, ceaſe before or after delivery.

Abortion and Miſcarriage; Uterine Hemorrhage, or Flooding. If not in their immediate, yet in their future conſequences, miſcarriages are much more fatal to puerperal women than appears in the London regiſters. Abortion or miſcarriage, or premature excluſion of the fœtus, may happen through every month of pregnancy. But the exact age of uterine embryos and abortions is, in ſome degree, conjectural. Before the ſeventeenth day after conception, its rudiments are not even viſible to the naked eye. The ſize of an abortion comprehending the fœtus, its membranes, waters and placenta, at the end of ſix weeks, does not exceed in bulk that of a pigeon's or hen's, and in three months a gooſe's egg. At the end of the fourth month its length is between four and five inches, and at the end of the ninth month between ſixteen and twenty-one inches; and its weight from ſix to ten pounds. Early miſcarriages between the third and fifth month, though not recorded in the burials, are, notwithſtanding, far more numerous than in the latter months; but are infinitely leſs hazardous to women. The mature abortives and ſtillborn, are alone thought deſerving of formal interment, and of notice in the regiſters. To carry a diminutive embryo, a Lilliputian in miniature, to a church-yard, and to bury it with funeral pomp and obſequies, would be ridiculous. In all probability, a very great majority of the regiſtered abortives and ſtillborn in London, had arrived at or near the full period of uterine maturity. Some miſcarriages are ſudden, with little or no warning, and with eaſe; others again are ſlow.

Uterine hemorrhage, or Floodings are ſeldom fatal to women before the two or three laſt months of pregnancy; the gradations of danger increaſing to the end of the ninth month, at which period the uterine blood veſſels are enlarged, and the hemorrhagick torrent is in proportion. The mouth of the womb alſo being then leſs diſtended than in ordinary parturition, is more difficultly forced open to expedite delivery. Floodings may at intervals, and ſome weeks precede natural parturition or miſcarriage; and after a temporary ceſſation, are prone to return on the ſlighteſt irregularity. Their danger is eſtimated from the quantity of blood, the ſuddenneſs of the torrent, and the debilitating effects on the mother; and if near the full period of geſtation from the abſence of labour pains. Uterine hemorrhages may occur not only in abortion and natural parturition, but alſo immediately, or ſoon after the birth of the infant, and extraction of the placenta; and are always alarming.

The

The predifpofing and occafional caufes of abortions and floodings are, frights, terror, anger, violent agitations of mind or body; ftrong mufcular exertions and efforts; external injuries, blows, falls, running, leaping, coughing, crying, fainting, hyftericks; plethora; errors in the non-naturals; impetuous flow of blood to the womb, falacity; too much amorous dalliance; too ftrait lacing and drefs; hot clofe rooms; foul air; difagreeable fmells; cravings not gratified; fpirituous liquors; abufe of emmenagogue, cathartick, and diuretick medicines; hardened feces and coftivenefs; piles; extreme irritability of the body and womb; weak hyfterical conftitution; weak difeafed fmall, contracted, not fufficiently dilatable womb; weaknefs of the uterine veffels from preceding abortion, irregular menftruation; poor blood; fluor albus; previous injuries during parturition; repetition from habit; the habitual tendency towards menftruation every month; hereditary; acute or chronic difeafes; morbid adhefion of the placenta, and alfo coalefcence with the womb from previous inflammation; partial feparation of the placenta; rupture of the veffels on the furface of the placenta; feparation of the falfe chorion from the womb; adhefion of the ovum or placenta to the neck of the womb: blights and difeafes of the fœtus, fcarcity of nourifhment in the womb, its violent efforts, monftrous fize; rupture of the navel ftring, a noofe formed upon it; long compreffion of the infant's head or navel ftring during parturition; injuries by the hands or inftruments of the accocheur; a dead fœtus.

Puerperal

Puerperal Convulsions may happen before, during, and after delivery. They resemble epilepsy, with froth at the mouth, distortion of the countenance and body; and are a much more terrific and frightful spectacle than hysterical and nervous spasms. In the advanced state of pregnancy, convulsions are still more dangerous, and, like the sudden impetuosity of a whirlwind, sometimes close the fatal scene; especially if at the same time a violent pain is felt at the stomach. The plethoric and robust are not exempt from this tremendous assailant; but the hysterical and delicate are the most frequent victims.

The predisposing and occasional causes of puerperal convulsions are morbid sensibility; profuse uterine hemorrhage; want of due quantity of blood; plethora; frights; low spirits; fear, dread, surprize, and sudden emotion and agitation of mind at this critical period; dead foetus.

Irregularity of the Lochia, comprehending excess, obstruction, and suppression. After delivery, there is generally a gush of red blood, from about a half to two pounds. The mother is then weak and infirm, from the fatigue and efforts of parturition; from the great evacuation and diminution of the womb and abdomen; from the loss of blood; from the agitatiton and anxiety of mind; and from the increased irritability: and women are then more than at any other time prone to fevers. In most cases the placenta is expelled in ten, twenty, or thirty minutes after the infant. Afterwards, the orifices of the uterine vessels continue to discharge

red

red blood, which gradually becomes thin and ſerous, and even in ſome degree purulent.

This diſcharge, named *Lochia*, is various in duration and quantity, from two to ten ounces daily, and, gradually decreaſing, in about ten or twenty days is dried up; nature having then reſtored the womb to its natural ſize: and at this ſtage, all immediate puerperal danger is eſcaped. Sometime there are great variations in the lochial duration in different women: in ſome, they ceaſe after a few days; in moſt, after two or three weeks; and in a few others, not until after one or two months: the duration and quantity being varied by climate, ſeaſon, conſtitution, mode of life, and ſtate of the breaſts. Lochial exceſs is determined more by the morbid and debilitating effects, than the abſolute quantity. Or in its conſequences it may more ſlowly ſap the pillars of health, and occaſion conſumption or dropſy. But obſtruction and ſuppreſſion of the lochia is much more frequent and dangerous than exceſs. Moſt of the uſual complaints after delivery, ſays Smellie, originate from obſtruction of the lochia, or of milk. Obſtruction is accompanied with pain of the back and loins, pudenda, and groins; heat, ſhivering, hard quick pulſe, reſtleſſneſs; ſometimes cholick and diarrhœa, and difficult oppreſſed reſpiration.

Inflammation of the Womb begins generally between the fourth and ninth day after delivery, and commonly with retention of the lochia: with fever, heat, acute ſenſibility and pain about the uterine region, irritation to urine and ſtools, colick, intenſe headach, ſtrong full pulſe. The whole, or different parts only, of the womb may be inflamed, whence the contiguous viſcera of the pelvis will be differently affected. Where the inflammation is not violent, the criſis is about the fourth or ſeventh day from the attack; but if ſevere, may be protracted to the ninth, eleventh, and fourteenth, and be then diſcuſſed with ſome ſenſible evacuation, by perſpiration and ſweat, by urine, diarrhœa, lochial diſcharge, or current of milk from the breaſts; or may terminate fatally in gangrene, delirium, and convulſions.

The prediſpoſing and occaſional cauſes of irregularity of the lochia, and of uterine inflammation, are, of exceſs, grumous clots of blood in the womb; violence done to the womb during parturition; retention of the placenta, or part of it; great weakneſs; paſſions of mind; a ſecond child; ſpaſm; repulſion of milk from the breaſts; too early and violent motion or walking about; diſeaſed ſtate of the womb; inverted womb; errors in food, drink, paſſions of mind, excretions, &c. Of obſtruction and ſuppreſſion; clots of blood in the vagina; cold admitted to the naked body, either externally or internally; cold rooms, cloaths, and drink; obſtructed perſpiration; impure air and cloſe heated rooms; paſſions of mind; hyſtericks; errors in the non-naturals, diarrhœa. Of inflammation of the womb, ſuppreſſion of the lochia; external violence; falls; rude extraction of the placenta; morbid adheſion of the placenta; miſcarriage; too tight bandages round the abdomen.

Puerperal

Puerperal Fever, or Peritonitis, commonly alledged to be peculiar to women after delivery, has been dignified by the moderns, from its danger and fatality, with a generic name: happily for the fair ſex, it does not often occur: ſometimes it is epidemic, from ſome unknown quality of the atmoſphere and ſeaſons; and in ſuch circumſtances a conſiderable number of puerperal women are afflicted at the ſame time. It generally attacks one or two days, but ſometimes a few hours after delivery; and rarely later than the ſixth day. The aſſault is ſudden and violent, with darting pains, and extreme tenderneſs in the abdomen, ſickneſs and vomiting of bile, and with prodigious proſtration of ſtrength and ſpirits. At the beginning, the ſymptoms and topical pains of the abdomen have an inflammatory appearance; but after a very few days the fever changes, undiſguiſedly, into the nervous and putrid type, and ſometimes with miliary eruption. Often neither the lochial diſcharge, nor the milk, are interrupted; and it has been obſerved to enſue even after eaſy labours. The puerperal fever will be affected and diverſified by different conſtitutions and temperaments, whether robuſt, plethoric, or delicate; by the quantity of the lochial diſcharge, the putrid atmoſphere in the ſick room, the medical treatment, the ſtate of the atmoſphere and ſeaſons, and morbid quality of the prevailing febrile epidemick. Between five and fifteen days terminates the event in recovery or death. It is always moſt fatal when moſt epidemick, and the ſooner it attacks after delivery. In ſome of our London hoſpitals, one half of the

the women ill of this fever have died; in others, one of seven.

The predisposing and occasional causes of the puerperal fever are, a peculiar noxious constitution of the atmosphere; errors in the non-naturals; anxiety of mind; hot cordial regimen; heated unventilated rooms after delivery, and impure air; hence miliary eruptions and profuse sweats. The immediate cause is generally ascribed to inflammation of the omentum, mesentery, or peritoneum. But it merits the most serious investigation, whether to employ the remedies accommodated to inflammatory, or to nervous and putrid fever. We know that purulency in the abdomen and thorax is likewise found in the putrid fever of the West Indies, in which the antiphlogistick course would be certain destruction.

After-Pains; *Weed*, *Milk-Fever*; *Inflammation of the Breasts*, are far less formidable foes than the preceding. After parturition, women are sometimes afflicted for some days with harrassing pains resembling colick. The causes are, the continued and sudden contraction of the womb towards its natural dimensions; fragments of the placenta or membranes, or of clotted blood in the womb; injuries done to the fibres of the womb during parturition; violent extension of the suspensory ligaments; inflammation and irritation of the womb, or its neck: tender state of the intestines; flatulence; flatulent food; suppression of the lochia; errors in the non-naturals; a second child. Weed, or ephemera, sometimes occurs from some errors in the non-naturals, and is the most simple and innocent

innocent ſpecies of tranſitory fever; reſembling an intermittent paroxiſm; and in the ſpace of a few hours, or at the utmoſt days, the fever diſappears.

During pregnancy and parturition the breaſts ſympathize greatly with the womb. The Milk-fever begins three or four days after delivery, with ſhivering and heat, pain, diſtention and throbbing of the breaſts; after twenty-four hours, commonly terminating by ſweat, diarrhœa, eruption of milk. In this puerperal ſtage, inflammation of one, but rarely of both breaſts, is a frequent affliction, varying in degree and ſeverity; and terminating by diſcuſſion, frequently by ſuppuration; ſometimes by ſcirrhus. The cauſes of this inflammation are, impetuous ruſh of milk; not ſuckling; obſtruction of milk in the breaſts or lactiferous tubes; ſuckling too ſoon; obſtructed lochia; cold and obſtructed perſpiration.

CHAP. XIV.

INFANT DISEASES every where furniſh a vaſt ſupply to the gloomy realms of Pluto; and this calamity is infinitely aggravated by the noxious atmoſphere of cities and towns. Out of four million of annual deaths in Europe, one million of theſe are under 1 year of age: and eight hundred thouſand more between 1 and 5 years: ſome of them from diſeaſes already, and others yet remaining to be deſcribed. At birth, an infant is not only uſhered into a new world, but every function of its frail body undergoes new and ſudden changes. From the human oven of 96 degrees of heat, it is launched into a variable climate of heat and cold. A new element of many thouſand pounds weight then preſſes upon the ſurface of its body. This atmoſpherick fluid, adulterated in cities with innumerable impurities and feculencies is drawn into its lungs: its diaphragm and muſcles of reſpiration then begin to act, the lungs expand, and reſpiration commences. The paſſage between the auricles of its heart and arterial duct are gradually cloſed; the ſphere of the circulation is extended; the whole current of blood in its frequent revolution hourly, paſſes through the lungs; the circulation through the navel-ſtring, and through which it had till then drawn its principal nouriſhment, inſtantly ceaſes: food, for the firſt time, begins to be taken in by its mouth; and the digeſtive, with all the numerous ſecretory and excretory organs, then begin to perform their different offices. The fetal brain is deſtitute of ideas; but inſtantly the tender creature is expoſed to ſounds, and in a few days to light: the bones at the ſuperior part of its head gape, and the brain is there defended by ſkin only; its head, abdomen, liver, and lymphatic glands, are large, and its extremities ſlender: its bones are little more than griſtles and cartilages; its muſcles are ſoft, flabby, and without ſwell or expreſſion: the greateſt part of its time is ſpent in a ſtate a ſtate of inactive vegetation: it is unable for ſeveral months to ſupport its own weight, or to take nouriſhment, and is then the moſt feeble and helpleſs of all the animal creation. With ſuch delicate machinery, it has ſoon to encounter pain and diſeaſe; the aſſaults of internal and external enemies; when its crazy beams and bolts are eaſily ſhook aſunder in the firſt ſtorm.

The acute diſeaſes of early infancy; that is, under two years of age (ſmall-pox, meaſles, and a few others excepted) are in the London regiſters, principally accumulated into two aggregate heaps, *Convulſions and Teething:* the former of which forms a dreary catalogue of aſtoniſhing magnitude in London funerals; amounting to nearly one third of the whole mortality in the metropolis. But convulſions and teething are terms too indefinite. Every infant diſeaſe, not immediately obvious to the ſenſes, is thruſt into theſe two articles by the ignorant reporters. If we conſider the term ſcientifically, convulſions, in multitudes of caſes, convey no more intelligence of the nature of the diſeaſe, than if they had ſaid the child died from want of breath.

Some adult mortality, but in all probability a very inconſiderable portion, is included in convulſions: infants are the principal victims. The convulſive liſt diminiſhes during the latter half of the preſent century; but to unravel the problem reſpecting convulſive increaſe or decreaſe, requires more elaborate inveſtigation than preceding calculators and criticks ſeem to have ſuſpected. It is neceſſary to contraſt the deaths by both convulſions and teething with the chriſtenings; for if more are born, more ſhould be

 expected

expected to die in infancy. We muſt alſo take cognizance of ſome other titles of London diſeaſes, particularly ſtoppage of the ſtomach, colick, and gripes, both which have been already under review. Beſides chryſoms and infants, an obſolete term, denoting the deaths in the firſt month after birth, is long exploded from the bills, and probably ingulfed in convulſions.

Let us examine, whether the collected obſervations of medical authors will not illuminate many dark and defective parts of the publick regiſters, reſpecting infant mortality. Infants are exempt from a multitude of the acute and chronic diſeaſes of adults: they rarely ſuffer ſo early in life from hereditary diſeaſes, cares, paſſions of mind, painful impulſes of retentive memory, ſevere ſtudy, intemperance, hard labour, the inclemency and viciſſitudes of the ſeaſons, and ſo on. The principal diſeaſes of infancy may be comprehended under the following: convulſions, inward ſpaſms and tetanus, colick, vomiting, acidity, indigeſtion, flatulence, diarrhœa and gripes, thruſh, dentition, hectic fever and atrophy, rickets, ſcald head, raſh, dropſy of the head and ſpine, inguinal ruptures; together with ſmall-pox, meaſles, hooping-cough, worms. Several of theſe diſeaſes are common to all ages, and have already been deſcribed under the reſpective titles; to which the reader muſt refer. We obſerve alſo in the Chart, that ſeveral infants are overlaid during the period of nurſing.

As infants cannot by ſpeech expreſs their pain, we are too often under the neceſſity to gueſs at their complaints by phyſiognomy, geſtures, and

dumb

dumb ſigns; theſe are principally manifeſted by nauſea, indigeſtion, vomiting, acidity, flatulence, refuſal of food, or the breaſt, diarrhœa and its different colour and conſiſtence, reſtleſſneſs, cries, ſhrieks, agitation and contraction of the lower extremities, diſturbed ſleep, injured reſpiration, cuticular eruptions, puſtules, and ulcers. In infancy the pulſe and urine are precarious ſymptoms.

The general cauſes of infant diſeaſes and mortality may be referred to the ſudden and violent changes after birth in its tender machinery; to weakneſs and injuries from tedious and laborious parturition; delivery before the end of the ninth month; hereditary debility; diſeaſed parents; foul air of cities; improper food and drink; ſcarcity of food and milk; ill formed nipples; the tongue tied or retracted; errors in quantity or quality of nutriment; too long continuance of vegetable and aceſcent food; foul ſtomach and inteſtines; acidity in its ſtomach: from errors of the mother or nurſe in food, drink, reſt, exerciſe, excretions, paſſions of mind, from ill temper, hyſtericks, addiction to raw ſpirituous liquors and drunkenneſs, diſeaſes, faſting too long before the infant ſucks; unwholeſome milk; adulterated milk and bread; neglect of cleanlineſs, and ſuffering the infant to lay too long in wet cloaths; inſufficient exerciſe, and alſo too violent agitation of the infant; the ligatures, bandages, and pins too tight, and tormenting the infant; improper poſitions and poſtures; cold cloathing and habitations, beds, and ſcarcity of fuel, eſpecially in northern regions, and in winter; defective or exceſſive excretions, and eſpecially by the anus; improper treatment and quackery of old women and nurſes, and other ſuch medicaſters, during its illneſs. It is but candid alſo to confeſs, that, in numerous inſtances, the cauſes of infantile maladies are not yet ſufficiently eſtabliſhed nor explained.

Convulſions, Inward Spaſms, and Tetanus. From the exquiſite tenderneſs and irritability of its frame, moſt diſeaſes of infants, when fatal, ſeem to terminate in ſpaſms, epilepſy, and convulſions; with which they are infinitely more afflicted than adults, and often endure better. Inward ſpaſms are amongſt the firſt of infantile maladies. The paroxiſms are uſhered in by ſome ſymptom of lethargy, by tremulous motion of the face and lips, and livid circle round the eyes and mouth, ſudden ſtartings of the muſcles, and ſtoppage of reſpiration, flatulence. By continuance, theſe ſpaſms often terminate in ſome of the following diſeaſes: hectic fever, thruſh, vomiting, diarrhœa and green feces, watery gripes, convulſions. Infants alſo are ſometimes ſubject to a locked jaw; which we have already noticed under Tetanus.

The prediſpoſing and occaſional cauſes of convulſions and inward ſpaſms are, fulneſs and foulneſs of the ſtomach and inteſtines; acrid ſtimulus of food, acidity, or bile, or inflammation in its ſtomach or inteſtines; general debility; compreſſion of the brain during parturition, hence mould ſhot, horſeſhoe head; water in the brain; teeth cutting the gums; paſſions and frights of the nurſe affecting her milk, or her drinking raw ſpirituous liquors; improper food of the nurſe or infant; premature repulſion of ſcald head,

head, excretion behind its ears, and cutaneous raſh. Laſtly, internal derangements in its crazy machinery. (See Colick and Diarrhœa.)

Dentition. It is probable that the mortality under this head is exaggerated enormouſly in the London regiſters, amounting there to one fifteenth part of the annual burials. Dentition uſually commences about ſix or ſeven months after birth; ſometimes not before ten, twelve, or eighteen months, and, in ſome extraordinary inſtances, not before two years of age. Theſe ſharp bones, in piercing the tender gums, more eſpecially if out of the regular ſucceſſion, often excite exquiſite pain, reſtleſſneſs, fever. But it is only in the firſt dentition, that is, under two years of age, that mortality enſues from this ſource: the fatal and moſt frequent tranſition is into convulſions.

Rickets. Notwithſtanding the omiſſion of ancient authors to diſcriminate this diſeaſe, we cannot believe but that, in this inſtance, the ſame cauſes would in all ages have produced the ſame effects. Rickets would ſeem by the London regiſters to decreaſe; for in our laſt group of fifteen years they ſhrink to 104; whereas in the thirty laſt years of the preceding century, ricketty deaths are numbered at 11,415. To what cauſe is this decreaſe to be aſcribed? Does it indicate more propriety in ſuckling and rearing of infants, or errors in the diſcrimination of diſeaſes? Rickets, one of the chronic diſeaſes, and affecting the ſolid props of the body, ſeldom commence before three, ſix, or nine months after birth, generally between nine months and two or three years of age, and ſeldom or ever after

after five. They begin with averſion to motion, decay of ſtrength and fleſh, tumid abdomen. The earlier rickets commence, they are more contumacious; and when chronic or fatal, are frequently accompanied with hectic fever: they may continue ſeveral years, and at length terminate in general bad health, atrophy, dropſy. Should they not be checked before the fifth, or at the utmoſt, the eighth year, irremediable deformity and crookedneſs of the bones, eſpecially of the lower extremities and ſpine, muſt enſue; which in females is often the cauſe of diſtorted pelvis, and difficult labours.

The prediſpoſing and occaſional cauſes of rickets are, hereditary; weak diſeaſed parents or nurſes; negligent nurſing; not ſufficient exerciſe nor cleanlineſs; improper diet and groſs food; worms; foul ſtomach and inteſtines; ſcrophulous obſtructed meſenteric and lymphatic glands; diſeaſed liver; general bad health, with hectic fever; various cauſes of atrophy; difficult dentition; faulty ſtate of oſſification; deficiency in the oſſious rudiments; faults in the organs of nutrition.

Thruſh. In the preceding century, *Canker* was often joined together in the London regiſters with Thruſh; but whether it ſhould be coupled with this or with gangrene, or with both, I cannot determine. Ulcerations and incruſtations of the tongue and mouth called Thruſh, is principally a diſeaſe of early infancy: it is likewiſe often a concomitant ſymptom of ſome febrile and acute diſeaſes of adults. It infeſts not the young alone, but alſo aged perſons, eſpecially in cold northern and moiſt climates, in damp ſituations,

ſituations, and in warm rainy ſeaſons. As an idiopathic diſeaſe of adults, it is rare in this iſland. The duration and event is various. If, after ſcaling off, the tenaceous incruſtations ſhould be ſucceſſively renewed, the diſeaſe may be protracted even to weeks; or may prove fatal in a ſhort ſpace.

Aged—" The race of man like leaves on trees are found,
Some green in youth, ſome withering on the ground."

So far the father of poetry. By ſome, old age is termed the ſecond ſtage of childhood. Dr. Short thinks, that aged in the London regiſters muſt denote thoſe advanced to near 70 and upwards: and of the indigent claſs of this deſcription, many of them, no doubt, inhabitants of parochial poorhouſes. But with reſpect to the dilapidation by time, much will depend on conſtitution, mode of life, and climate: ſome are worn out at 60, whilſt others at 70 are healthy and vigorous. About one tenth or twelfth part of the annual mortality of Europe, that is, about 400,000, conſiſts of aged. Many reaſons, however, induce me to believe, that not one half of thoſe reported as dying of age, do yet, in reality, founder by gradual decay, but are cut off by ſome of the diſeaſes already deſcribed; which occurring in theſe latter ſtages of life, are confounded with the ruins of time. The immortal phyſiologiſt, Haller, ſays, " rara mors ſenlis " eſt, tamen aliqua: ſæpius in beſtiis;" who expire from a univerſal debility of all the nerves and

and muſcles, voluntary and involuntary, and eſpecially of the heart. We have excellent treatiſes, ancient and modern, on old age; but medicinally, we are yet defective in ſpecific diſcrimination and excellence. What has been propoſed by that great philoſopher, Lord Verulam, of confining the vital ſpirit, is more ingenious than practical: and in ſeveral reſpects is diſſonant from ſound philoſophy. For by age the ſolids and ſanguineous canals become rigid, ſtraitened, and cloſed; the earthy parts increaſe; the nerves, ſenſes, internal and external, the muſcles, heart, and inteſtinal canal become more inſenſible, callous, torpid; the humours are diminiſhed and corrupted, together with the perſpiration; and with an increaſing decay of muſcular ſtrength and of the heart, the tottering fabrick at length glides into the grave.

CHAP. XV.

A Miſcellaneous group of diſeaſes are here aſſociated: ſeveral of them unconnected in ſymptom, cauſe, or cure: others are of exotic origin, and tranſplanted amongſt us: moſt of this cutaneous claſs are ſlow and chronic. Mankind left expoſed, without defence or remedy, againſt even this ſmall morbid hoſt, would ſoon be ſenſible of the calamities and

ſcourge

ſcourge of medicinal ignorance: and they would be leſs ſurprized at the incorporation of medicine with divine worſhip in ancient times.

Venereal Diſeaſe. In the laſt 30 years of the preceding century 2360 deaths are recorded under French pox, in the London bills; and even at this day, the chart of diſeaſes demonſtrates its fatality to be infinitely greater than profeſſional men could ſuſpect. Three hundred years have not altogether elapſed ſince the diſcovery of America, and the importation of the venereal diſeaſe into the old world. Before the diſcovery of its antidote, mercury, and in ſome inferior degree of the native Indian remedy, the decoction of guiacum, Europe was alarmed with univerſal conſternation at the rapid inroads of this diſeaſe: multitudes, of all ranks, periſhed in lingering torture, under its corroding ulcers, preſenting before death hideous ſpectacles of cadaverous corruption and deformity.

It would, in this diſeaſe, be ridiculous to inſpect hoſpital regiſters, for the purpoſe of either aſcertaining the ages wherein venereal ravages prevail, or the proportion of cured and incurable. Its ravages cannot be infancy, nor in adoleſcence, nor in the decline of life. The mereſt ſmatterer in medicine knows the infallible remedy and cure; except that in the application to particular caſes, ſome more judgment and dexterity is neceſſary. The multitudes who now periſh in theſe battles of Venus, are ſo many ſacrifices either to negligence or to indigence; or to the groſſeſt ignorance and empiriciſm of licenced murderers. There is no other diſeaſe wherein profeſſed quackery is ſo generally reſorted to, or wherein its decoys are ſo pernicious to the community. The great majority of theſe victims to ſeduction, pleaſure, and neceſſity, are in all probability amongſt the ſwarm of wretched and unfortunate female proſtitutes; and in the male ſex amongſt the lower orders: for in thoſe of leſs ſtraitened circumſtances, a ſmall bribe to the ſearchers would conjure venereal mortality into ſores or ulcers, or into conſumptions. Beſides, were we to add to venereal carnage the ſhattered conſtitutions of young men of all ranks, in conſequence of theſe wounds and ſcars, it would appear an object of ſufficient magnitude to attract the attention, interpoſition, and regulation of the legiſlature. In every metropolis, more eſpecially amongſt the unmarried, and profligate, and in armies and navies, it is without doubt, much more fatal to the community.

There are two diſtinct genera, or ſpecies, of the venereal diſeaſe; the local gonorrhœa, and what is called confirmed pox. The gonorrhœa generally begins a few days after infection with oozing of mucus from the male urethra, or the female vagina, and dyſury; the latter of which is not ſo troubleſome in females. The lues venerea confirmata, or ſyphilis, commonly begins with either one or more ulcerations of the penis, or vagina; or with inflammation in the glands of the groin, called bubo; which may either originate from previous ulcer or without it. Theſe are the two uſual and ſlight appearances of gonorrhœa, and of confirmed pox, when the infection is firſt applied to the genitals; and frequently theſe two genera are complicated. But

in

in both genera, from various cauſes, originating from the virulence of the diſeaſe, the intemperance of the patient, or miſmanagement of his medical pilot, many adventitious and aggravated ſymptoms are ſuperadded; in number and ſeverity varying in different perſons: ſeveral of them, when violent and precipitate, requiring ſpeedy alleviation; and often to be treated as ſeparate diſeaſes.

In the malign train of gonorrhœa are violent inflammation and conſtriction of the prepuce, before or behind the glans, or phymoſis, and paraphymoſis; dyſury, ſtrangury, priapiſm; painful and inflamed teſticles; ſcirrhous and indurated teſticles; chronic gleet; ſtricture, caruncles, and obſtructions in the urethra. Confirmed pox, in its inveterate and chronic ſtages, contaminates the whole conſtitution; erodes the genitals, or anus; aſcends to the throat, and excites callous ulceration and dilapidation in the uvula, tonſils, fauces, palate, noſe; hence hoarſe, guttural voice, fetid breath: the patient is variouſly tormented with chronic gnawing pains in the head, legs, ſhoulders, and hard bones, which are exaſperated in bed; with cutaneous eruptions on different parts of the face, trunk, or extremities, and dry, ſcaly, humid, ulcerated, red, yellow, or purple; with ophthalmy; with nodes and tumour of the forehead, exoſtoſes and caries of the bones; atrophy. Chronic warts about the genitals and anus, and called by different names, porri, cryſtæ, condylomata, rhagades, thymi, moræ; are generally innocuous.

The causes of gonorrhœa and pox are, Infection by contact with the genitals: or the pox, when inveterate, may be communicated by the mouth and nipples; by drinking out of the same vessels, by touching any diseased or ulcerated part. When inoculated by suction, it begins first in the mouth or nipples.

Scurvy. True scurvy is seldom or ever mentioned by any writer, before the long voyages, first began three centuries ago by the moderns; that is, on the discovery of the passage to Asia by the south cape of Africa; and the discovery of America. Then, in consequence of living long on salted and gross diet, and the want of fresh vegetables or fruits, together with their ignorance of the cause and cure, this disease made dreadful havock amongst naval squadrons, and the other busy hive employed in nautical commerce. The ancient navigators, who seldom ventured out of sight of land, or capes; and who probably were not under the necessity of subsisting long on salted food, do not appear to have suffered by, nor even to have known, the disease. Hippocrates is supposed slightly to allude to scurvy, under the name of large spleen; accompanied also with spungy putrid gums, and offensive breath: it is also, though indistinctly, noticed by Pliny, as affecting a Roman army encamped on the banks of the Rhine.

Through all the northern kingdoms of Europe, particularly in the winter season, and in Holland, amongst those who fed chiefly on salted fish and gross diet; who drank bad waters, and dwelt either in morasses, or near the sea coasts, and were exposed to cold and moisture, scurvy

ſcurvy in the two laſt centuries made cruel ravages. Several armies and beſieged garriſons in Germany, intercluded from freſh vegetables; and numbers of the new ſettlers in the northern colonies of America, and who were in nearly the ſame predicament, were cut off by the ſcurvy. The North Americans were at laſt taught by the Baltickers and Swedes the ſovereign benefit of ſubſtituting ſpruce beer, when freſh vegetables cannot be found. The induſtrious Dutch made drains and canals to carry off water, and truſted the reſt of the cure or prevention to pickled cabbages or ſour crout. In the northern parts of Ruſſia, where ſcurvy is very univerſal, they found a particular acidulated bread and ſour drink, powerfully to reſiſt this diſeaſe.

By theſe and other precautions, the ſcurvy is now much leſs formidable on land; but at ſea no other, the nervous and putrid fever excepted, is ſo inimical to navigators. On that element it is yet the ſecondary devouring monſter and tyrant. In the firſt voyages of our Eaſt India Company's ſhips, nearly one fourth of the crews died at ſea. Nautical records teem with tragical narratives of ſcorbutic ravages. But at preſent, the cauſes, the effectual antidotes, and the cure, are ſo well known, that the greateſt part of the lives now loſt by ſcurvy at ſea, are either ſacrificed to groſs negligence, or to impolitic and inhuman economy. The temperature of ſea air is more equal than that on land: and that it is not pernicious, we have an undoubted proof in one of the late Captain Cooke's voyages; wherein, with a company of

118 men, during a voyage of three years, and through all climates, from 52 degrees north to 71 ſouth, he loſt only one man by ſickneſs.

From 1671 to 1686, the deaths, by ſcurvy, are in the London bills 9,451; but in the ſucceeding fifteen years, decreaſe to 569 only; and throughout the preſent century, continue progreſſively on the declenſion. Even of this trifling number, what proportion was engendered at ſea, or whether they all died of genuine ſcurvy, I cannot decide. The theory of the laſt century imputed many diſeaſes to this ſpecific cacoethes, as they called it; which would have ſome influence on the ſearchers reports. In London, the lodgings are now warm and dry, and the people in general tolerably well cloathed: animal meat is eat freſh; vegetables, though perhaps not univerſally conſumed in ſufficient quantity, are certainly in much greater abundance than formerly: beer, fermented liquors, and tea, are alſo drank by all ranks. All theſe, in conjunction with exerciſe, powerfully reſiſt the tendency to ſcorbutic corruption. I am inclined to ſuſpect that in the reports it was often confounded with Leproſy.

The progreſſive gradations and virulence of ſcurvy, are diſtinguiſhed under the three following ſtages: pale, ſickly, and bloated countenance, laſſitude, averſion to motion, debility, on any exerciſe. But the cardinal ſymptom is red, ſpungy, enlarged gums, from which, on being rubbed, blood iſſues, and the teeth begin to looſen; the breath and urine are fetid; and, by degrees, bruiſes and black ſpots are ſeen in various parts, eſpecially the legs. In the ſecond

more

more aggravated ſtage, the tendons at the hams begin to contract and ſwell; there are pains in different parts; diſpoſition to ſalivation, and hemorrhages from the gums and noſe, with increaſed debility and proneneſs to ſyncope. In the laſt and moſt inveterate ſtages, putrid ulcers are formed, particularly in the legs, which are ſwelled and enlarged; or old cicatrices of former ulcers are diſſolved, and again break out, from which iſſue a ſanious and fetid diſcharge; and within them is generated fungous fleſh, in conſiſtence reſembling a bullock's liver. Throughout there is no fever; nor is the diſeaſe contagious; neither are the appetite and ſenſes conſiderably impaired, except that there is great deſpondency and melancholy.

The prediſpoſing and occaſional cauſes of ſcurvy are cold and moiſture, and ſubſiſting long on dried, ſmoked ſalted fleſh meat or fiſh, without vegetables, or theſe in ſmall quantity; putrid, and alſo groſs diet difficultly digeſted, not perſpirable; corrupt ſtagnant water; low marſhy damp ſituations; cold ſituations; the winter ſeaſon of northern climates: wet cold cloaths, beds, houſes; inſufficient or ſuppreſſed perſpiration, hence the corrupted animal juices are not carried off; indolence, ſedentary life, confinement, dejection of mind, melancholy; bad health; impurities of the blood; diſeaſes and obſtruction of the ſpleen, liver, and vena porta.

Scrofula, Struma, King's Evil. In the laſt thirty years of the preceding century, the mortality by evil is only 2,126, in the London bills; and throughout the preſent century continues decreaſing. This, however, is a very partial representation of its fatality, which in its consequence is far more destructive. The disease seldom appears under two years of age; commonly between three and seven, and sometimes not until near puberty; after which its evolution and first appearance is very rare. The children of fair hair, rosy cheeks, smooth skin, soft delicate complexion and temperament, are more obnoxious to scrofula than those of an opposite temperament. It is sometimes introduced by a tumid upper lip, and chop in the middle of it; at other times the first appearance is oval moveable tumours in the lymphatic glands of the neck, under the chin or below the ears. These are various in size from a walnut to an egg, or larger, and often continue inert one, two, or more years, and without pain, until they tend towards suppuration. At length there is some fluctuation, ulceration, and exudation of viscid serum, but no concocted pus, and tardy cicatrization. In this way there is a succession of tumours and ulcers during several years; some cicatrizing, and others breaking out.

Commonly after four or five years, or towards puberty, the cervical ulcers finally close, leaving behind indelible scars. This entailed alloy is often the source of bad health. Sometimes the eyes or eyelids are particularly afflicted with scrofulous ophthalmy. In other cases it excites tumours, deep seated abscess, anchylosis, and caries in various joints of the elbow, fingers, knees, feet; or stubborn ulcers in different parts: and still more deleterious consequences ensue from scrofulous glands of the lungs or mesentery terminating

terminating in phthiſis, or hectick. Some nations more than others, are afflicted with ſcroſula. I have read that it is not frequent in tropical climates; and it is not contagious.

The prediſpoſing and occaſional cauſes are hereditary: diſeaſes of the lymphatic glands; conſequence of ſmall pox. Whether it is more prevalent in ſome countries than others from the air, water, diet, or other cauſes, is not yet aſcertained.

Leproſy. The abſolute mortality in the London bills, by this diſeaſe, is almoſt undeſerving of notice. A conſiderable part of the Moſaical code, politically and medicinally, is pointed againſt this diſguſting cutaneous diſeaſe; but it is now, in a great degree, eradicated and worn out of Europe. After the Cruſades, in the twelfth century, Europe was overſpread with this hideous judaical ſcurf, imported from Paleſtine. Lazarettoes for the confinement of the unclean, and for the performance of a leprous quarantine, were then numerous in many kingdoms: in France alone there were two thouſand. At preſent, in the cold northern iſland, Iceland, a ſort of leproſy is congenial to the natives, from their diet, climate, and mode of life. And in the hiſtory of the late diſcoveries in the Pacific Ocean, we read of a leprous ſcurf infeſting the natives, from their exceſſive indulgence in a hot ſpice amongſt their food. In our iſland, at this day, a conſiderable number are afflicted with a chronic cutaneous ſcurf; but greatly inferior in virulence to the Aſiatic leproſy.

The ancient and modern writers diſtinguiſh leproſy under two ſpecies, or gradations, the Lepra Græcorum, and the Lepra Arabum, or Elephantiaſis. The impetigo or lichen, herpes, and what is vulgarly, but improperly, denominated the endemic land ſcurvy in this iſland, ſeem merely branches of leproſy; and it is for the cure of this, certainly not of genuine ſcurvy, that we have ſuch a proſtitution and inundation of empirical noſtrums, eſpecially of the mercurial kind: this laſt ſpecies is alſo frequently periodical. In the Lepra Græcorum, the ſkin in one or in ſeveral parts is hard, rough, prurient, with ſmall red puſtules coaleſcing into cluſters of different dimenſions; and ſooner or later, exudations of ſerum corroſive, viſcid, from which are formed ſqualid incruſtations: in ſome, the ſkin in the inſide of the hands and fingers is parted into fiſſures. In other caſes, the ſkin, partially or generally, is only dry, rough, prurient, diſcharging large quantities of ſcales, which are ſhed in the bed like handfuls of bran, and with the cuticle the nails often fall off. In the inveterate ſtages, the whole ſurface of the body is polluted with this abominable fetid ſcurf, accompanied with headach, reſtleſſneſs, and derangement of the corporeal functions. The Elephantiaſis is the moſt diſguſting and inveterate of all diſeaſes; but this exotic genus is now very rarely ſeen in any part of Europe: the ſkin is thickened and rough, with fetid incruſtation, ulceration, deſquamation, fiſſures, together with interſperſed tubercles, livid, hard, painful, deforming the face, neck, and other parts of the ſurface; exciting reſtleſſneſs, hectic, emaciation

ciation, cachexy, dyſpepſy, hoarſeneſs, depilation, and a long train of collateral evils. Every ſpecies of leproſy is ſlow, chronic, contumacious; but at preſent, in moſt caſes, the European leproſy at length yields to regimen and remedies; whereas the Aſiatic and African is often incurable.

Amongſt theſe offenſive cutaneous maladies we may aſſociate the morbus pediculoſus, a diſeaſe very rare, but of which I have ſeen and cured ſeveral caſes. Plutarch mentions Scylla, the Roman dictator, and ſeveral other conſpicuous names of antiquity, as deſtroyed by this loathſome cachexy.

The prediſpoſing and occaſional cauſes of leproſy are often obſcure: ſome are hereditary; infection; obſtruction or raſh repulſion of hemorrhoides, menſes, old ulcers, ſcald head; dregs of intermittent fever or ſmall-pox; impure blood; general cachexy; diſeaſes of the cutaneous glands; cold and moiſt climate, or local habitation; obſtructed perſpiration; diſeaſes of the liver, and bile; impure groſs diet and waters; exceſs of hot ſpices and ſeaſoning in diet, or of ſalted, ſmoaked, rancid fleſh or fiſh, and of bacon, oatmeal, cheeſe, &c. poor diet, with poverty and its conſequences; ſometimes ſymptomatic in the venereal diſeaſe; ſcurvy.

Itch, pſora. Some few deaths appear in the London regiſters from this cutaneous and infectious diſeaſe. It is a frequent complaint in camps, navies, hoſpitals, poor houſes, jails; amongſt ſome trades more than others, and more amongſt the indigent and ſqualid than the affluent:

affluent: but is rarely dangerous to life, or even health, unleſs improperly or raſhly repelled It uſually begins on the inſide of the wriſts and fingers with ſmall red prurient puſtules more or leſs general; ſpreading often, if not prevented, to the ſides, hams, legs, and other parts of the body, the face excepted, exciting inceſſant heat and irritation to ſcratch; hence laniation, ulcerations, ſcabs, and incruſtations. The immediate cauſes are, ſubcutaneous animalcules: the remote cauſes may be deduced from thoſe of leproſy.

Achores, Favus, Cruſta lactea, Tinea Capitis, Plica Polonica. Moſt of theſe ſeem only to differ in gradation, and the parts which they affect. They denote pruriency, ulcerations, glutinous exudations, ſcabs, and fetid incruſtations, on the hairy ſcalp, or the forehead, varying in colour, conſiſtence, thickneſs, extent, diſcharge. They are moſt frequent in infancy, and often ſalutary. The cauſes are variouſly aſcribed, to exceſs of pituita in early years; unwholeſome milk; diſeaſe of the ſebaceous glands; infection; and perhaps to ſome of the ſources of leproſy. —The Plica Polonica was originally imported from Aſia into Poland, where it is now principally predominant. In it the hairs of the head are entangled by a viſcid exudation into inextricable ropes and clots of tenaceous paſte. It is infectious, and not peculiar to any age or ſex. Some weeks or months previous to this capillary diſcharge, the conſtitution and functions of the internal and external ſenſes are greatly deranged, with headach and wandering pains:

hence

hence it proves critical and ſalutary, and not dangerous to life, but often chronic.

Gutta Roſacea. Carbuncles, pimples, and tetters on the face, are frequent complaints of both ſexes, and principally amongſt adults. Their origin is various, hereditary; impure blood, or acrid ſerum; local diſeaſe of the ſebaceous glands; drunkenneſs; ſurfeits; acrid, ſalted, or groſs diet; moiſt cold climate, or local habitation; obſtructed perſpiration; imprudent repulſion of natural evacuations; paints; critical, ſalutary; periodical; ſymptomatic in venereal, ſcorbutick, and ſome other diſeaſes.

Yaws, a morbid exotic, infectious, and if not peculiar to, at leaſt moſt frequent amongſt the Africans, and the exported negroes to European colonies: in its mature ſtages, indicated by puſtules, in which are generated red fungous fleſh, in ſize, colour, and ſhape, reſembling a raſpberry or mulberry; appearing about the genitals, anus, and face, and varying in number.

CHAP. XVI.

MURDER, robbery, ſedition, and war, are amongſt the principal political caſualties, chronic diſtempers, fevers, inflammations, and frenzies of every nation. From the neceſſary ſeverities, or the tyrannical exerciſe of juriſprudence;

risprudence; and from the mad projects of ambition, avarice, or caprice of princes and ministers, an immense carnage is made amongst the human species, but principally amongst the male sex, and those in the prime of life.

Murdered. During the last 30 years of the preceding century, the murdered in the London registers are 432: but of late years this dreadful crime seems to decrease. Whether this is to be ascribed to the streets being better lighted and watched, to less savageness and brutality, not only amongst the lower class, but even amongst thieves and robbers, to fewer swords being worn, to the Foundling Hospital, for the reception of illegitimate deserted infants, or to these and other causes, I submit to the reader. Some great cities of the Continent are far more infamous for assassination and murder than the British metropolis. It would be both curious and useful to ascertain the proportion destroyed by duelling, by the brutal exercise of boxing, and by other accidental rencounters; and as influenced by different governments, laws, and gradations of civilization.

Self-Murder. A peculiar gloomy passion and propensity of the English, as they alledge on the Continent, has increased in the present century; and greatly exceeds the murdered. During the last 30 years of the preceding century, those marked as hanged, drowned, and made away with themselves, are only 556; whereas now they are doubled. And it is generally believed, that the total amount is concealed in the London registers, whereby a considerable emolument is derived by the coroners of the county from

from the relations of the deceaſed, in order to their procurement of a different report; ſuch as found dead, ſuddenly, drowned, lunatick. This violent and ſhocking diſſolution is principally amongſt adults, and both the ſexes, but probably is more predominant amongſt males. The ancient Romans were notorious for the ſame propenſity and crime; it was indeed incorporated with their legiſlative and moral code. To illuſtrate the malady and its cauſes would require an intricate digreſſion into national character, conſtitution, paſſions, manners, diet, climate, &c. Its immediate cauſes have a ſtrong affinity with thoſe of inſanity, which have been already diſcuſſed and demonſtrated.

Drowned. The number drowned in London, during the laſt 30 years of the preceding century, were 2182. It is obvious, that in maritime and commercial iſlands, and in the vicinity of navigable rivers, ſuch accidents will be more frequent than in continents; and more ſo amongſt male adults and youths. When we behold the multitude of ſeamen, watermen, and paſſengers on the river Thames, and of perſons bathing in ſummer, many diſaſters of this ſort muſt be expected, and will be inevitable. Beſides, not a few of the drowned are caſes of lunacy or premeditated deſtruction. Drowned perſons, formerly, were often ſuſpended by the legs, or laid in a prone or bent poſture, with the head downward, from an erroneous idea, that the lungs and ſtomach were filled with water. With more judgment and ſucceſs the moderns, firſt the Dutch, and afterwards the Engliſh and other nations, direct heat, inceſſant friction, ſtimulants

lants to the nofe and lower inteftines, as volatile falts, and tobacco fumes, and warm air to be blown into the lungs. We have modern records of recovery, in all the intervals, from 3 to 30 minutes after fubmerfion; and in fome of thefe cafes fymptoms of life did not appear until after one or two hours perfeverance in thefe proceffes for the revival of the circulation and vital powers. I believe, however, there are no authentic inftances of recovery after being buried only a quarter of an hour under water; more efpecially in the winter feafon. In thefe cafes, as in the plague and feveral other difeafes and cafualties, found political wifdom fhould direct the principal attention to the prevention, and not to the forlorn hope of cure. The Greeks and and Romans did not confider the cleanlinefs and health of their fubjects beneath their notice, but provided them with convenient baths: the young and inexperienced, or thofe in hazard of finking, would be rendered ftill more fecure by the occafional affiftance of corks.

Executed, banifhed, and imprifoned. In afcertaining the numbers executed, particularly, the London bills of mortality are fhamefully erroneous and defective. As I thought it a cafualty of infinite importance to be exactly ftated and recorded, I made numerous efforts to procure authentic information, by fucceffively and repeatedly waiting upon the Keeper of Newgate, the Clerk of the Arraigns, the Clerk of the Peace for the County, the Town-Clerk of London, the Sheriff's office of London, and the Secretary of State's. Throughout this inquiry I was every where treated with liberality and

and urbanity; and where there was any proſpect of information, was permitted acceſs to the records. But, to my aſtoniſhment and mortification, I could not find any veſtige of records of executions in London before 1754. Theſe were in the Clerk of Arraigns office, but were buried in a heap of extraneous law rubbiſh; to extract which, the Clerk told me, would require three entire days for myſelf and one of his aſſiſtants. I called twice at the Old Bailey, anxious to undertake this taſk, however laborious; but it ſo happened, that at both times they were full of buſineſs in the office, and could not ſpare time, nor even room for my inquiry. By other means, I have diſcovered part of the truth. (*Vid.* CHART.)

The two firſt columns, from 1732 to 1762, are formed from an average of executions, during twenty-two years of that interval, by Sir Theodore Janſen, Chamberlain of London. The laſt column, of fifteen years, is formed from an average of the laſt ſeven years, with which Mr. Akerman politely furniſhed me, from his books. In conſequence of the riots and conflagration in 1780, his records were all conſumed, and do not include that year, wherein there was a notorious glut of executions. During the ſeven years beginning with 1781, the executed in Mr. Akerman's books were 439. But every one knows that there are two theatres, a great and a ſmall one, appropriated for human ſlaughter in this metropolis; theſe are Tyburn, now removed to Newgate; and for the large Borough of Southwark, Kennington Common. I took a low average of the executions in the latter, allotting three

three annually, to the two firſt columns, and ſix to the laſt column, and added the whole together. Amongſt the London malefactors there are a few extraneous pirates, whoſe crimes were committed on the ſea, but are cognizable in the Admiralty Court of the metropolis.

Two thirds, probably, of all thoſe capitally condemned, are afterwads pardoned. Few, comparatively, of the executed have committed murder, not one in twenty; moſt of the reſt are for robbery, theft, and frauds of various kinds: the analyſis, proportions, and gradations of which, I leave to the profeſſors of juriſprudence. Many more, it is true, are reported as murdered in the bills of mortality: but theſe are not caſes of premeditated and malicious homicide, and are ſoftened into manſlaughter on trial. Nineteen out of twenty of the executed are males; and by far the greateſt proportion between eighteen and forty years of age. What is the proportion of London executions to the whole nation, is a problem which perhaps our judges cannot unravel. Vice and executions are univerſally more prevalent in every metropolis: but there is reaſon to believe, that at preſent the executions throughout Britain and Ireland, are double or treble to thoſe of London. The comparative population is as ten million to ſeven hundred thouſand. If they are treble, then 4000 are executed every fifteen years in the two iſlands; and 26,000 in a century: and both the diſeaſe and panacea are rapidly increaſing. Five or ſix times this number are, in the ſame period, tranſported to diſtant regions, and partly alſo loſt to the community, together with their blighted procreation. Were the reſt of Europe to give equal employment to their executioners and goalers, the total amount is eaſily aſcertained by a common rule.

We are ſtruck with horror even on reading in hiſtory of the ſavage juriſprudence, cuſtoms, and butchery of mankind in ancient times; ſuch as the ſanguinary codes of Draco and other regal monſters; the ſacrifices to idols; the martyrs to gloomy fanaticiſm; the brutal ſpectacles of the Romans. But I doubt whether, in the moſt flagitious and facinorous ages of Rome, the Tarpeian rock was beſmeared with the blood of ſuch a multitude of human victims; or that in any part of the globe, from London to the Antipodes, out of an equal proportion of mankind, there are ſo many ſacrifices annually made to violated juriſprudence; and to the modern idol, property and money.

Beſides the political patients doomed to the radical cure, or extermination, by the executioner, if we may credit one of our beſt writers, they are a mere handful compared to thoſe who are conſigned to a ſlow and lingering death. Theſe formulæ, in the juridical pharmacopœa, may be compared to the hot iron and cautery of the coarſe empiricks of antiquity; with which they outrageouſly and indiſcriminately tortured their patients. Dr. Johnſon, in one of his excellent eſſays in the Rambler, againſt perpetual impriſonment for debt, calculates, that half a million of mankind are deſtroyed in a century in the priſons of Great Britain, by the complicated horror of confinement and ſorrow, by famine, filth, and diſeaſe; and to theſe I would

 add

add ſuicide. I am inclined, however, to believe, that Dr. Johnſon's computation is exaggerated, by at leaſt four hundred thouſand. By far the largeſt proportion of theſe are unfortunate ſacrifices to poverty and misfortunes, and to the callous vindictiveneſs of avarice: perhaps not a few of them cruſhed by the enormous publick taxations and accumulated exactions, from the induſtry of individuals during the preſent century: all of them are adults, and by far the greateſt proportion males. It would not diſgrace the chriſtianity or humanity of our legiſlators and lawyers, were they to reviſe their catechiſm and breviary of juriſprudence, both as affecting life and liberty: or, throwing religion and humanity to one ſide, let the queſtion be tried by commercial ſcales; and, like the Venetian Jew, let human fleſh be eſtimated in ounces, pounds, and pence, with brutes, metals, and chattels! Is debt the only heinous offence for which Britons are to be deprived of liberty and life, without even a trial by jury to diſcriminate between deliberate fraud, and accidental calamity? The eſtabliſhed aphoriſm in juriſprudence, "that from the *ſeverity* of puniſhments "even crimes are not leſs frequent" is equally applicable to this inſtability, and involuntary reverſe of fortune.

Wars. Since the invention of gunpowder, and the introduction of fire arms into modern tacticks, fewer are killed than in ancient times, when battles were chiefly decided by grappling in cloſe fight; and when ſlavery was the fate of the vanquiſhed: fewer alſo, comparatively, are killed at ſea than in land engagements; and for obvious

obvious reaſons, infinitely fewer in the aggregate on ſea than on land: it is alſo obvious, that theſe martial ſacrifices are confined to the male ſex, and principally within the procreative age between 20 and 60, when millions, every century, of mankind are ſwept away with the ſtock and future progeny. But whether we regard ancient or modern times, ſickneſs and diſeaſe are immenſely more formidable enemies, both at land and ſea, than the weapons of the enemy: by theſe morbid foes the ſinews of military ſtrength are cut, the ſcale of defeat and victory turned, and armies, fleets, and nations rapidly overwhelmed in calamity and ruin. The greateſt part of mankind are yet to learn, that medicine is an indiſpenſible knowlege of every legiſlator and general who is ambitious of pre-eminence, or is prompted by a conſcientious diſcharge of duty. The ancient and modern authors on the elements and ſublime principles of war, moſt of whom I have peruſed, are ſhamefully deficient in this eſſential department of military ſteerage. With what abſurd puerilities and pernicious precepts is even that eminent modern author, Marſhal Saxe, disfigured, when he ſeriouſly recommends, from the example of the Romans, vinegar as the grand panacea to preſerve troops healthy. The predominant noxious diſeaſes of armies and navies are few in number, and have already been deſcribed: they are fevers and dyſentery, conſumption, peripneumony, rheumatiſm, ſcurvy, dropſy, venereal diſeaſe; excluſive of thoſe in common with all mankind of ſimilar ages, and in other reſpects in ſomewhat parallel ſituations. Fractures, external inflammation, gangrene, ruptures, yet remain undiſcuſſed. It ſhould alſo be obſerved, that the ſeaſon of greateſt ſickneſs and mortality, at leaſt in armies, will be, during the tumult of military operations, which are uſually in ſummer; and conſequently the mortality of this ſeaſon will be the reverſe to that of mankind in a ſtate of domeſtick tranquillity; and the many hardſhips and inconveniences attending a ſtate of warfare will alſo aggravate the diſeaſes and mortality.

I mean, from the earlieſt authentick hiſtories of war, that is, from Moſes and Homer, to deſcend in chronological order through the hiſtories of the Greeks and Romans, and their numerous enemies; and through the numerous domeſtick and foreign conflicts of modern nations, down to the preſent time, both by land and ſea; to contraſt the proportion of killed and of diſeaſes and mortality, their ebb and inundation. From this general ſurvey I flatter myſelf to be enabled to draw inferences, and eſtabliſh propoſitions of ſuperlative political and military moment. On this ſubject a very elaborate and learned treatiſe will ſoon be publiſhed by a friend of mine, Dr. Millar, from which the publick, and the author of theſe obſervations, will derive important inſtruction.

To the READER.

WE are obliged to cut off the remainder of our comments, amounting to fifty pages, which would have compleated, on our plan, the univerſal ſurvey of the diſeaſes, caſualties, and mortality of the human ſpecies. The index aſcertains the omiſſions. Under Gangrene I ſhould have diſcriminated the ages, cauſes, mortality, and as originating from ſpontaneous corruption, external injuries, or ſurgical operations. Under Fractures I ſhould have gauged the cures and miſcarriages after the trepan and amputation; diſcriminating, at the ſame time, between ſudden accidents and chronic diſeaſes. This is a moſt important part of military ſurgery, and in a great meaſure unexplored. Through abſceſs, ulcers, and ſores, of which there is ſuch an overflow in our hoſpitals; and throughout cancer and lithotomy likewiſe, I ſhould have applied the ſure and certain teſt of medical arithmetick.

CHAP. XVII.

OF the Institution of the London Bills of Births, Mortality, and Diseases; their Defects, besides those already pointed out; important and easy Improvements recommended; and applicable to every metropolis and kingdom.

We shall now, with all possible brevity, enquire into the degrees of credibility and stability of the mathematical and medical data, furnished from the bills of mortality. The births genealogies, procreation, multiplication, and deaths, of those few miracles of longevity, from Adam to Noah; from Noah's descendants down to Abraham, Moses, and Christ, are recorded in scripture: some chapters of Genesis are plain registers of births and mortality. The male Israelites, above twenty years of age, were, at distant intervals, mustered and numbered by Moses and his successors; and in a few uncommon pestilences, the devastation is ascertained in the Jewish history. The descent and pedigree of kings, and other great men, have also been kept in most nations, who had made any progress in civilization: but general annual registers of births, diseases, and deaths, are modern establishments, and were unknown to the ancients. At the same time the aggregate mortality would be discovered by numbering of the people, which was annually practised by the Greeks and Romans, and several other nations of antiquity: by this they were enabled to ascertain

certain the number fit to bear arms in cafes of emergency.

On the continent of Europe, regifters were inftituted fifty or a hundred years before their introduction into England. In 1538, exact records of weddings, chriftenings, and burials, were firft ordered by the King and council, to be kept in every parifh church of England, by either the vicar or curate. But this order was very negligently obeyed in many parifhes, until 1559, when, to prevent regifters from rotting in damp churches, they were directed to be written on parchment. At firft, they feem, both in Germany and England, to have been defigned to prove the birth, death, and defcent of individuals, and the right of inheritance in property or lands. In 1592, a year of peftilence, bills of mortality for London were inftituted; but were difcontinued until 1603, another year of peftilential defolation; which was the only diftemper then taken notice of in the printed reports. In 1626, the different difeafes and cafualties of thofe who died in London, together with the diftinction of the fexes, were added and publifhed; and in 1728, the different ages of the dead were ordered to be fpecified in the London bills. Upon firft eftablifhing the diftinction of difeafes and cafualties in the bills of the Britifh metropolis, the primary intention feems to have been, to diftinguifh the numbers deftroyed by the plague, and to detect concealed murders.

Public records of births and mortality are now partly become the rules of political arithmetic: but unfortunately for politicians, calculators of annuities, and phyſicians, they are yet every where far too incorrect and incomplete. Regiſters of diſeaſes and deaths in London are entruſted to old women, two of whom are nominated in each pariſh, hence called Pariſh Searchers, and who conſider, the ultimatum of their commiſſion is merely to prevent private funerals and concealed murder. The whole buſineſs in London is conducted in the following manner: Upon either being ſent for to inſpect a corpſe, or on hearing the bell toll, and inſpecting the books kept in the different churches, the ſearchers are appriſed from whence notice has been ſent of a death, in order that a grave may be opened. The two parochial matrons then, whoſe induſtry is ſtimulated by a ſmall fee on each corpſe, and whoſe report is neceſſary previous to interment, ſet out to examine that no violence is committed upon the dead, of which they have taken an official oath to make true declaration, and afterwards negligently enquire from the relations the name of the diſeaſe, adding the age and ſex: or ſometimes they are ſtopped in the hall, and diſmiſſed without any ſcrutiny. Theſe records, together with the chriſtenings, in the latter of which the ſearchers have no concern, are depoſited with the reſpective clerks of each pariſh church, and by the clerks the chriſtenings of the eſtabliſhed church, and the burials in their reſpective parochial church-yards alone, are carried once every week to a general hall in the city: on the following day the weekly bill, comprehending theſe partial returns, is printed and publiſhed; and at the end of the year a general bill, in which all the weekly returns are consolidated.

The law ordains, that every person who dies in the registered parishes of London, Westminster, and Southwark, is to be inspected by two parish searchers, and reported to the parish clerk, who then grants his certificate for the interment: or, if the corpse is carried away to a different parish of the metropolis for interment, the searchers report, and the clerk's certificate, are equally necessary; otherwise that parish where the corpse is buried is liable to a fine. This process was originally intended to detect the plague, and concealed murders; in both which respects, during the present century, the parish clerks and the searchers have been almost useless. There is now no plague to detect; there are very few murders, and they are always proclaimed by some other means. Even in the preceding century, when the plague raged in London, the searchers report was rarely trusted without a physician or surgeon attending, to prevent mistakes.

Notwithstanding this ceremony of inspection by the searchers, and of making their reports to the parish clerk, it does not hence follow, that the clerk makes the return of the death to the general hall, *unless the corpse is buried in his own ground, or parochial church-yard*. If the corpse is carried to any dissenting ground, and to various other places of sepulture not within the bills, the death and disease is so much waste paper, and is never heard of amongst the burials. But if the corpse is carried to a different parish, together with a certificate, and such burying ground

ground is regiſtered within the bills, then the death and diſeaſe is returned to the hall by the clerk of that pariſh where the corpſe is interred.

I made it my buſineſs to viſit, and to converſe with a variety of pariſh clerks in this metropolis, moſt of whom agreed with me, that, beſides radical defects in the chriſtenings and burials, there were many other groſs omiſſions. One inſtance I ſhall mention, and many more might be collected. The pariſh clerk of Bethnal-green, in which are alſo three private madhouſes, made no return to the general hall, during the year 1780, of either births or burials, and in the preceding year he returned only four burials: whereas in former years, this pariſh alone annually returned from three to five hundred burials. I was aſſured, that the company of pariſh clerks in their corporate capacity, even if willing, have no power of compulſion over any of their refractory and negligent members, to make regular and correct returns: it ſeems almoſt optional. It is obvious what flagrant diſcordance and error this muſt occaſion in various calculations.

Excluſive of groſs miſmanagement and error from ſearchers and pariſh clerks, there are other inherent defects in the London regiſters, both of burials and births. They comprehend the births alone of thoſe belonging to the eſtabliſhed church, and the burials of ſuch only who are interred in the regiſtered parochial church-yards. Jews, Quakers, Papiſts, Proteſtant Diſſenters of various ſects, are not included in the annual chriſtenings; and great numbers of their burials, and of the burying-places, not only of the diſſenting,

ſenting, but likewiſe of the eſtabliſhed church, are omitted: of the former 32, and of the latter 35, according to Short's Liſt. Maitland, 1729, (ſee his Hiſtory of London) diſcovered 181 religious congregations, whoſe chriſtenings were not publiſhed, and 63 burying-places in and contiguous to the metropolis, wherein 3038 were annually buried, but excluded from the regiſters. The large modern and populous pariſhes of Pancras and Mary-le-bone, in one of which alſo ſtands the Foundling Hoſpital, are omitted in the annual bills. Six hundred abortive and ſtillborn, who have arrived at an age thought deſerving of funeral, are added to the annual deaths, but omitted in the liſt of births; as are alſo many young infants who die before baptiſm.

I ſaid, that very few of the chriſtenings of the diſſenting ſects in London were included in the public regiſters; but ſeveral of them are buried according to the formalities, or at leaſt in the cemeteries of the eſtabliſhed church; which muſt unnaturally magnify the comparative liſt of deaths. Another defect in the burials is, that numbers are carried into the country who are not accounted for: it is agreed that ſeveral hundreds more are annually carried out of than are brought into London for interment. Moſt of the nobility and gentry are removed from London, after death, to their family ſeats. Dr. Price calculates the preſent annual deficiency in the London burials at 6000; and of the births ſomewhat greater; neither of which are brought to account in the regiſters.

The

The following is an average, which I have formed from the London bills of christenings and burials:

London Bills at a Medium annually.

Years.		Christenings.		Burials.
From 1671 to 1681	—	12,325	—	19,144
1681 to 1691	—	14,439	—	22,363
1691 to 1700	—	14,938	—	20,770
1700 to 1710	—	15,623	—	21,461
1711 to 1720	—	17,111	—	23,990
1721 to 1730	—	18,203	—	27,522
1731 to 1740	—	16,831	—	26,492
1741 to 1750	—	14,457	—	25,351
1751 to 1759	—	15,119	—	21,080
1759 to 1768	—	15,710	—	22,956
1770 to 1780	—	17,218	—	21,000

A TABLE of Thirty Years, formed from the London Bills, beginning with 1728, and ending with 1757; shewing the Total Number of Deaths and comparative Decrease in this Period, at every Age.

Years of Age.			Died.
Under	—	2	272903
From 2	to	5	64745
5	—	10	25912
10	—	20	22891
20	—	30	58474
30	—	40	71502
40	—	50	73258
50	—	60	59872
60	—	70	47269
70	—	80	33679
80	—	90	16948
90	—	100	2496
100	—	138	242
Total Deaths in this Period, at all Ages,			750,191

The

The parifhes, but not all the burial grounds in thefe parifhes, now included within the London bills of mortality, amount to 147: of which there are 97 within the old city walls; 17 without the walls, but within the city liberties; 23 out parifhes in Middlefex and Surry; and 10 out parifhes in the city and liberties of Weftminfter. All the 97 parifhes within the walls have not, for many years paft, at a medium, buried 2000 annually: fome of them do not make a return of a fingle burial in feveral years. We may name feveral parifhes without the walls, any two of which united, return a number of annual deaths equal to the 97 parifhes within the walls. In collecting and conducting the bills of thefe parifhes, there is a rabble of 294 female fearchers, and 147 parifh clerks.

To render the returns of births, chriftenings, weddings and burials in London complete, the clergyman of every religious fect fhould be compelled, by law, to make monthly returns of their chriftenings and weddings to the neareft parochial church. All the church-yards and burying grounds hitherto excluded from the bills, together with the parifhes of Pancras, Mary-le-bone, and all the other modern additions and population to London, fhould likewife be comprehended in the regifters; together with the numerous villages and excrefcences of the metropolis, within feven miles of its circumference. There appears, at prefent, no neceffity to return weekly bills from the different parifhes to the general hall. This was originally intended to warn the London inhabitants of the numbers deftroyed by the plague, and the infected

fected parishes. Monthly returns would be sufficient, united and printed in one general annual bill, in which the monthly christenings, weddings, and mortality should be distinguished; in order to point out the seasons most prolifick, or most noxious; to mark the reigning diseases, and the hurricanes and monsoons of mortality.

The christenings should specify the name, sex, twins or tergemini, the illegitimate if known, and the religious sect. The weddings should discriminate the place of abode of the parties, the names and ages of each pair; whether first, second, or third marriages, and on which side; whether natives or foreigners, and the religious sect.

In infancy, and the early part of life, when the tide of devastation is strong and rapid, the mortality should be measured in shorter intervals. The first year from birth should be divided into interstices, from birth to six months, when teething commences; from six months to one year; from one to two; two to three; three to four; four to five; five to ten; ten to twenty; and so on to one hundred and upwards. Exclusive of abortions and stillborn, those who die in the first month before baptism, and of course cannot be included in the christenings, should be distinguished, in order to determine more accurately the amount of the abortives and of the births. Separate columns should be assigned for the name of the disease or casualty; for the cause, if known; and the duration of the affliction. Annexed to each disease should be the numbers dying at different ages of that

malady.

malady. Males grown up to maturity who die, ſhould be diſtinguiſhed either as married, widowers, or bachelors; and females alſo of this deſcription, either as married, widows, or virgins. Thoſe carried out of London, or into it, for interment; the parochial children who die at nurſe in the vicinity of the metropolis; the rank, profeſſion, or trade, and whether native or foreigner, ſhould all appear in the general annual report in ſeparate columns. The annual reports of all the hoſpitals, diſpenſaries, parochial poorhouſes, priſons, and of the executed, ſhould alſo be made to the hall, and included in the general annual regiſter.

There are often objections and ſcruples to apply effectual remedies, or radical cures, to ancient inſtitutions, however defective and inadequate. There certainly is no neceſſity for ſuch a cumbrous complex machinery, or multitude of pariſh ſearchers and clerks, for conducting the London bills. Indeed they might probably be all diſpenſed with. The reports of the relations of the deceaſed, or of the pariſh officers, to the curate of the different churches, would perhaps anſwer every purpoſe; and the perquiſites would be a conſiderable addition to the clerical pittance. I mean, however, only to offer a ſimple, eaſy, and unexceptionable palliative; which is, to appoint a phyſician to ſuperintend the general hall, and the reports of births, burials, and diſeaſes: and the whole to be ſubjected to the inſpection of a committee of the Medical College, or of the Royal Society, or of both. This would give authenticity and reſpectability to the regiſters. In ancient Rome, the regiſtering

registering of the number of the people was committed to the most high and sacred dignity in the state, the Censor.

From such a rich mine, and treasury of medical and political facts, the most important and beneficial information would be derived; the increase or decrease of deaths, marriages, and births; the annual waste of the metropolis; the health, mortality, the diseases most fatal, their growth or declension; the effects of diet, drink, and medical practice; of metropolitan jurisprudence, and also of metropolitan charitable donations and institutions. Calculators of annuities, reversions, survivorships, insurances, of the conditional tenure of property in lands or money, on lives; together with public political loans, tontines, and annuities of various descriptions, would then be supplied with certain, instead of disputable data: at present this alone is a prodigious article of traffick and commerce in this country: much litigation and expence respecting births and deaths, and the right to inheritance, would also be prevented. In a word, an immense variety of most interesting medical and political propositions, which are entangled in intricacy and obscurity, would, by this means, be evolved, and indisputably demonstrated.

Besides, the progressive improvements in the prevention and cure of diseases must make considerable changes in tables of mortality and calculation: those formed in the preceding century for London, would differ from the present: and the succeeding century, probably, will be still more different. There is yet no possibility to reduce

reduce human mortality to that exact menſuration and revolution, by which aſtronomers have proved the great lunar and terreſtrial cycles to be regulated. The ſale of the improved Bills, making, according to my arrangement, about twelve different tables, would defray any additional expence. Whatever Plato may alledge to the contrary, the uſeful and practical is much preferable to the mere contemplative philoſophy. Or as Plutarch expreſſes it, "Knowledge ſhould be "converted into action, and not be conſidered "as a uſeleſs fund of talk."

It is alſo moſt devoutly to be wiſhed, for the health, comfort, and decency of the metropolis, that all, or at leaſt the majority of the burying grounds, were ordered to be formed in ſome dry ſpots of ground at the different extremities of the city; and that the dead were more detached from the living. No one whoſe curioſity for information has led him to theſe melancholy wrecks of human vanity, and to behold the yawning mouths of ſepulchres, can reflect without pain and aſtoniſhment, on the manner in which between twenty and thirty thouſand corpſes are annually crammed into various holes, corners, public thoroughfares, and churches of this city. Nor can theſe cadaverous exhalations fail to pollute the air, and to engender diſeaſes. Let the clerical revenue ariſing from graves be transferred to the new cemeteries.

CHAP. XVIII.

WE ſhall conclude, by pointing out the moſt celebrated treatiſes on human propagation, exiſtence, mortality, and morbid devaſtation, by ſeveral philoſophers. Graunt, ſomewhat later than the middle of the laſt century, firſt wrote a treatiſe on the London bills of births and mortality, and was followed ſoon after by Petty, King, and Davenant. The preſent century has produced ſeveral treatiſes on this ſubject; of which the moſt celebrated are Dr. Halley's; De Moivre's Treatiſes on Annuities and Chances; Suſmilch's Calculations; Simpſon's Select Exerciſes; ſome Eſſays in the Philoſophical Tranſactions; Dr. Jurin on the Small-Pox *only*; Dr. Short's Obſervations on various Bills of Mortality; M. Meſſance; Dr. Price's Eſſays, the Archimedes in annuitant and reverſionary calculation; Birch's Collection of the London Bills of Mortality to 1759; Dr. Percival's Eſſays; Dr. Millar's Calculations reſpecting the Diſeaſes of Great Britain, and Military Diſeaſes; and Dr. Robinſon's, reſpecting Maritime Diſeaſes. Some collateral information may be gleaned from thoſe excellent political and commercial writers, all of whom have adopted the numerical ſyſtem, Neckar, Hertzberg and Zimmerman.

This volume being ſo favourably received, I propoſe to conclude with a ſecond, on Therapeuticks, or the prevention and cure of the diſeaſes of of the human ſpecies. This will include the Materia Medica in the moſt extenſive ſenſe, and all the numerous collateral auxiliaries of medicine; together with dieteticks and drinks: the different ſyſtems of nurſing and education, ancient and modern: the different national inſtitutions and regulations for the culture and commerce of medicine, with the motly multitude, licenſed and unlicenſed, employed in exerciſing this divine art: the numerous publick inſtitutions, both domeſtick and military, devoted to the miſeries and diſeaſes of the indigent: and on each of theſe topicks the uſes, abuſes, defects, and errors.

Reſpecting one of the inſtitutions in London, for the ſmall-pox and inoculation, I have already, in a detached treatiſe, proved, that the principles upon which it is founded and ſupported are, in many reſpects, fundamentally erroneous and deluſive. One hoſpital, or one hundred hoſpitals in London, wherein none under ſeven years of age are inoculated, never can effect any conſiderable diminution of mortality by that diſeaſe, whoſe ravages amongſt the native progeny of London, and probably of every other great metropolis, are under ſeven years of age, as five to one greater than through all the remaining ſtages of life included.

F I N I S.